ARTHRITIS MEDICINES A–Z

ARTHRITIS MEDICINES A–Z

A Doctor's Guide to Today's Most Commonly Prescribed Arthritis Drugs

C. Michael Stein, M.D.

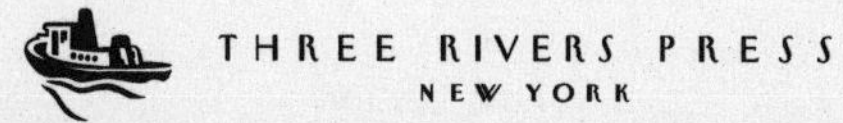

Published by Three Rivers Press, New York, New York
Member of the Crown Publishing Group.

Random House, Inc.
New York, Toronto, London, Sydney, Auckland
www.randomhouse.com

Printed in the United States of America

Design by Rhea Braunstein

Library of Congress Cataloging-in-Publication Data
Stein, C. Michael (Charles Michael)
Arthritis medicines A–Z : A Doctor's Guide to Today's Most Commonly Prescribed Arthritis Drugs / by C. Michael Stein.
p. cm.
1. Anti-inflammatory agents—Handbooks, manuals, etc.
2. Arthritis—Chemotherapy—Handbooks, manuals, etc.
RM405.S74 2000
616.7'22061—dc21
00-037432

ISBN 0-609-80507-X (pbk.)

10 9 8 7 6 5 4 3 2 1

First Edition

**This book is dedicated
to my patients
and my teachers.**

Publisher's Note

This book is intended to provide educational material to the public about common medicines that are used to treat arthritis and arthritis-related problems. It is not complete or exhaustive. It is not intended to substitute for any aspect of medical care. The choice of medicines, their doses, and instructions as to how each medicine should be used must be determined by the readers' physicians. Readers should work with their physicians to optimize their medical care and should not alter their medical care based on information provided in this book.

CONTENTS

INTRODUCTION

WHY I WROTE THIS BOOK

Arthritis is a common problem whose treatment can seem complicated. I wrote this book for people who have arthritis or an arthritis-related problem and for their families, to help them make sense of their arthritis medicines. You will find information about the various treatments for arthritis, the choices available, and how to make the most of your medicines.

People with arthritis are confused by the many drugs on the market. They look for information about their arthritis medicines but have trouble finding reliable and useful information that they understand. What they hear or read about arthritis treatment is often wrong, frightening, or confusing. In my office I realized that people were asking the same questions over and over again. Here are my answers to those questions.

No matter what anyone tells you (or tries to sell you), there are no cures for most types of arthritis. This book does not promise any miracle cures. What I do promise to do is teach you about the single biggest advance in the treatment of arthritis: using medicines effectively. I focus on prescription medicines—an area that has been neglected as interest has shifted to herbs, diets, and natural remedies. Recently, perhaps because of interest stimulated by new drugs, people have rediscovered prescription medicines, recognizing that they really work. This book teaches you about those medicines.

Thank goodness people don't always agree. My opinions are fairly mainstream, and your physician might have different opinions. Don't change your treatment because of something you have read, in this book or anywhere else, without first speaking to your physician.

GETTING INFORMATION ABOUT ARTHRITIS TREATMENT CAN BE A PROBLEM

Starting treatment for arthritis can confuse you and seem frightening because there are so many drugs and they all seem to have horrible side effects. I have learned that people, even those who seem very tough on the outside, often have problems dealing with their arthritis and its treatment. It is not easy to get useful information about arthritis medicines. Doctors often seem too busy, and if you do ask them something, it is difficult to remember exactly what they said after you have left the office. Some people go to the *Physicians' Desk Reference* (PDR), a thick medical reference book, to look up their medicines. The information in books such as the PDR is accurate, but it is not framed very well. An example will show you what I mean.

If swimming pools were medicines, no one would swim.

If a swimming pool were a drug that you looked up in a medical reference book, you would find something like this:

"Swimming pools may cause fatal side effects such as drowning and spinal cord injuries as well as other serious problems such as broken bones, sinusitis, ear infections, eye infections, irritant conjunctivitis, meningitis, diarrhea, fungal skin infections, and sunburn. Use of swimming pools has been associated with various skin cancers." You would certainly be afraid of swimming pools if you looked them up and read this, but your common sense tells you that swimming pools are really fairly safe, provided that you can swim and don't do reckless things such as dive into the shallow end. A long list of possible problems for swimming pools—or your medicines—is not helpful if it is not tempered by common sense. In *Arthritis Medicines A–Z,* you will find facts and a common-sense approach to arthritis medicines.

Caught in the web.

After looking in big reference books, the next place most people go for information is the Internet. You can find a lot of information about arthritis treatment on the various web sites out there. But unlimited access to unlimited information can also be a problem. Some of the information is accurate, but some of it isn't. It's hard enough trying to figure out which information to believe, not to mention deciding what applies to you and your type of arthritis. Looking for information about a drug shouldn't leave you paralyzed with fear or confused with information-overload—rather, the information should be accurate and organized so that it's helpful. Using this book, you will be able to judge the quality of information that you get from the web, and you will be able to use it rather than be caught up in it.

HOW TO USE *ARTHRITIS MEDICINES A–Z*

The A–Z Formulary contains the information about common arthritis medicines that I would like my own patients to have.

Finding your medicines is easy. Each drug is listed alphabetically under what is known as the generic name. Drugs have two kinds of names—generic names and brand names. Brand and generic names are similar to the way we name groceries. For example, ketchup would be the generic name that covers Heinz and Hunt's and all the many different brands of ketchup you can buy. One generic drug is often sold under many brand names, but all the brands contain exactly the same generic drug. Having many different brand names for the same drug can get confusing. Using one generic name that covers all the different brands that contain the same drug makes things simpler. It doesn't matter if you know only the brand names of your medicines. Most common brand names are listed in the A–Z Formulary in italics. You can look up your medicine by its brand name and find out the generic name. Under the generic listing the following aspects of the drugs are discussed:

Brand Names

Here you will find common brand names for this drug. Sometimes, particularly for common drugs such as aspirin or acetaminophen, there are too many brand names to list. Often, after drugs have been on the market for a while, more brands become available. The manufacturer chooses the brand name, but the generic name always stays the same.

Sometimes Called

When people speak about some drugs, they sometimes use an abbreviated or unofficial name. This section gives you those names so that you can understand which drug is being referred to.

Drug Family

This section tells you which family a drug belongs to. The information is useful because drugs in the same family tend to have the same effects, good or bad. That means you can get a rough idea of how effective a drug can be and what side effects it may have simply by knowing which family it belongs to.

Families of Arthritis Problems Prescribed For

Here you will find which arthritis-related problems a drug is used for. It will include uses approved by the Food and Drug Administration (FDA) as well as other uses for which there is evidence that the drug can be helpful. Arthritis-related illnesses do not always fit into neat slots. So, particularly if you have an unusual problem, you can end up on a treatment that is "proven" or "unproven" to a greater or lesser degree. Most rheumatologists are as practical as plumbers. They try to figure out what the problem is and try to fix it. Don't be alarmed if you are on a medicine (or combination of medicines) that has not been approved by the FDA for your particular problem.

How It Works

This section tells you how each arthritis medicine works. This can be useful since arthritis medicines that work in different ways are sometimes combined.

Avoid

In some people the risk of side effects from a particular medicine is high, and they are not usually treated with this drug.

This section tells you who should generally avoid a particular drug.

Regarding pregnancy: Some drugs are thought to be safe in pregnancy, and some are not. For most drugs, the information about risks in pregnancy isn't much good because the drugs have not been tested in pregnant women. The information provided by manufacturers is often not very helpful. For most drugs they say something like, "This drug is not recommended for use in pregnancy and should not be used unless the benefits are thought to outweigh the risks." Deciding how to treat arthritis in pregnancy is a very individual decision and depends on your problem, the medicines you are taking, and your feelings. If there is a well-known problem with a drug in pregnancy, I will usually mention it in the Avoid or Take Precautions sections, but because decisions about treatment in pregnancy are so individual, if you become pregnant, or plan to become pregnant, you should discuss with your physician what medicines you can and cannot take.

There are four important things you should remember about medicines and pregnancy:

- The time when medicines are most likely to harm the unborn baby is in the first weeks or months, when you might not even know you are pregnant. So if you are taking regular medicines and want to become pregnant, it is much better to discuss this with your doctor so that you plan the pregnancy, and any changes that might be needed in your treatment, *before* you try to become pregnant, rather than to just let it happen.
- If you become pregnant unexpectedly, talk to your doctor about this *immediately*.
- Physicians try to keep the medicines a woman takes during pregnancy to a minimum. For particular problems,

however, a pregnant woman might need to take medicines. The decision to use any medicine in pregnancy is made after weighing the likely results of the mother going untreated against the possible risks to the unborn baby. Many kinds of arthritis problems can be treated during pregnancy with drugs that seldom cause problems for the baby. Many pregnant women are treated for different types of arthritis and have healthy babies.

- Tobacco and alcohol, which we don't always think of as drugs, can have harmful effects on the baby. Don't smoke or drink alcohol if you are pregnant.

Take Precautions

You can decrease your risk of side effects by taking the simple precautions listed in this section.

Side Effects

All drugs can have some side effects in some people. Here you will find which side effects occur, how often they occur, and which can be serious.

Common side effects happen in 10 percent or more of people.
Less common side effects happen in 1 percent to 10 percent of people.
Rare side effects happen in 1 percent or less of people.

All men (and women) are not equal when it comes to side effects.

How often side effects happen and how severe they are vary from drug to drug and from person to person. Things that change the risk of side effects are the drug itself, the person taking the drug, and the problem being treated. Some drugs cause more side effects than others. Some people, because of their age, kidney or liver problems, allergies, other medicines that they are taking, or because they smoke or drink alcohol, can respond differently to medicines. Some illnesses affect the way drugs act. For example, people with psoriasis seem to have liver side effects from methotrexate more often than do people with rheumatoid arthritis. Fortunately—and unfortunately—every person is different. Some side effects are predictable, and others that we don't understand very well are not.

Predicting the unpredictable.

Side effects from drugs are often divided into two big groups.

Predictable side effects: These are side effects that can be predicted from what we know the drug does. In other words, a drug can have too strong an effect. For example, blood thinners (anticoagulants) are taken to prevent blood clots from forming, but if their effect is too strong, someone can bleed. Sometimes these side effects happen because someone is more sensitive to a particular effect of a drug, sometimes they happen because too much of a drug stays in the body, and sometimes they happen because of some other health problem. For example, someone who has diabetes can have worse diabetes after taking a corticosteroid drug like prednisone. We can decrease the risk from predictable side effects of drugs if we keep in mind the things that can increase problems with a particular drug in a particular person. The Take Precautions, Important Information, and Interactions With Other Drugs sections give you this information. If you know what makes the predictable side effects of a drug more likely, you can often take precautions that will decrease your risk.

Idiosyncratic side effects: This is a fancy way of saying that we haven't worked out why these side effects happen in some people. Idiosyncratic side effects, for example allergies, usually cannot be predicted or avoided, but if you are aware of them you can minimize any harm by taking action early or avoiding certain drugs that you know you are allergic to. If you are allergic to a drug you could develop a rash or, if you have a serious allergy, your tongue and face could swell and you could have trouble breathing. Side effects like nausea or vomiting are not usually caused by an allergy. Many people who have had a side effect like nausea after taking a narcotic painkiller say that they are allergic to that painkiller. That is not really correct. They have experienced a side effect that happens fairly often with that family of drugs.

Interactions with Other Drugs

When two medicines are given together, this can affect how one, or both, works. It can also change the risk of side effects.

- Some combinations of drugs work well together and are used to get a better response.
- Some combinations of drugs increase side effects and are usually avoided.
- Some combinations of drugs are used together, but because they have effects on each other, your physician might need to change their doses or monitor their effects more closely to avoid problems.

Important Information

This section highlights key information about the drug that I think is important for you to know.

Common Dose Sizes

Common tablet or capsule sizes that are available are listed.

Usual Adult Doses

These are the average doses prescribed for average adults. Remember, some people might need smaller doses and others might need larger doses. This is because different people are more or less sensitive to a particular drug and because different people clear the drug from their bodies at different speeds.

Comments

One of my teachers, Dr. Ted Pincus, says that treating arthritis is similar to baking a cake. Different people use different recipes to make the same type of cake, such as, say, a chocolate cake. Even if they all use exactly the same recipe, different people end up with very different cakes. You will find that not all doctors treat arthritis in exactly the same way. In the Comments section you will find my opinions about a drug or family of drugs. My opinions are fairly mainstream and are based on clinical studies published in the medical literature and on my experience treating patients. There are many unanswered questions in rheumatology, and experts can have different opinions. I like to keep an open mind and look at the hard evidence. I would like you to do the same.

IMPORTANT POINTS TO REMEMBER

- You are in charge of your treatment. Information that is inaccurate or confusing can harm your treatment. Information that is accurate and easy to understand will improve your treatment.
- Don't take medicines if you are pregnant without first speaking to your doctor.

- Don't change the dose of your medicines or the type of medicines you are taking based on what you read here or anywhere else. First discuss it with your doctor.
- Remember that medicines are only part of the treatment for arthritis. Exercise, physical therapy, surgery, and a positive attitude can also be very important.

FORMULARY
A–Z

ACETAMINOPHEN

Brand Names

Acephen, Aceta, Apacet, Panadol, Tylenol, and many others.

Sometimes Called

Acetaminophen is one of the few drugs that has a different generic name in different countries. In the United Kingdom and some other countries, the generic name is paracetamol.

Drug Family

Acetaminophen is an analgesic (painkiller). Acetaminophen is not a nonsteroidal anti-inflammatory drug (NSAID).

Families of Arthritis Problems Prescribed For

Acetaminophen is used for mild to moderate pain, whatever the cause. It also lowers fever, but does not decrease inflammation. Acetaminophen, because it does not cause stomach ulcers, is the drug most experts recommend should be tried first for pain caused by osteoarthritis.

How It Works

No one knows for certain how acetaminophen works. Acetaminophen may decrease the formation of chemicals called prostaglandins in the brain.

Avoid

Do not take acetaminophen if you are allergic to it.

Take Precautions

• Do not drink alcohol while you are taking acetaminophen because it increases the risk of liver problems. Fasting may also increase the risk of liver damage. The maximum dose of acetaminophen that is safe in most adults, a total dose of 4 g a day (equivalent to eight 500 mg tablets), may not be safe in people who are drinking alcohol or who are not eating regularly. Talk to your physician if these apply to you.

• The maximum dose of acetaminophen that is safe in most adults, a total dose of 4 g a day (equivalent to eight 500 mg tablets), may not be safe in people who already have a liver problem. Talk to your physician if this applies to you.

• Acetaminophen in overdose can cause serious, and sometimes fatal, liver damage. Keep acetaminophen away from children.

Side Effects

Acetaminophen, in recommended doses, is a very safe drug and seldom causes side effects.

Rare: Allergy and rash are rare. Liver damage is rare if recommended doses are used, but has occurred in a few people—usually people who have been drinking alcohol and taking acetaminophen. Liver damage caused by acetaminophen usually occurs after an overdose of the drug. The dose of acetaminophen that can cause serious overdose problems is close to the dose that is used to treat pain.

There is a possibility that taking acetaminophen regularly for a long time may, over years, cause kidney damage in a few people. This is controversial. In fact, acetaminophen, because it is so safe, is one of the painkillers most often used for people who already have kidney damage.

Interactions with Other Drugs

Alcohol, barbiturates such as phenobarbitone (*Barbita*), and isoniazid (*INH*): These drugs can increase the risk of liver damage from acetaminophen.

Warfarin (*Coumadin*): Acetaminophen, in a dose of more than 2 g a day, increases the anticoagulant (anti–blood clotting) effect of warfarin in some people. If you are taking warfarin to prevent blood clots and start taking acetaminophen regularly, you may need to have your blood monitored more frequently than usual, and your dose of warfarin may need to be changed.

Important Information

- Don't take more than the prescribed dose of acetaminophen.
- Don't take additional over-the-counter or prescription medications that contain acetaminophen. Many painkillers, both over-the-counter and prescription ones, contain acetaminophen. So if you are already taking acetaminophen, make sure that any additional painkillers you take do not push your total dose of acetaminophen up to more than 3 or 4 g a day.
- Don't drink alcohol while you are taking acetaminophen.
- Acetaminophen is dangerous in overdose. Keep it away from children.

Common Dose Sizes

Capsule and Tablet: 325 mg and 500 mg (the 500 mg dose size is sometimes called "extra-strength").

Usual Adult Doses

The usual dose of acetaminophen in healthy adults is 1 to 4 g a day, divided into three or four doses spread out over twenty-four hours. Do not ever take a total dose of more than 3 to 4 g a day (equivalent to six to eight of the 500 mg extra-strength tablets in one day). Even this dose may be too high for some people (see Take Precautions).

Comments

Acetaminophen is an effective and popular painkiller that is in most of our medicine cabinets at home. What many people don't realize is that for some people with osteoarthritis, acetaminophen is as effective as a nonsteroidal anti-inflammatory drug (NSAID) for controlling their joint pain. Acetaminophen and NSAIDs are different families of drugs. Nonsteroidal anti-inflammatory drugs, a mouthful that is abbreviated to NSAIDs (pronounced "*n*-sayds"), decrease pain and inflammation. The advantage of acetaminophen above NSAIDs is that it does not cause stomach ulcers. Acetaminophen causes fewer side effects than NSAIDs, so I usually try acetaminophen first for osteoarthritis.

Some people with osteoarthritis do well on acetaminophen, but it does not suit everyone. Some people add an occasional dose of an NSAID when their pain is bad, and others find that an NSAID works better for their pain than acetaminophen does. That is fine. If you have osteoarthritis and you find that acetaminophen and an NSAID are equally helpful for your pain, then acetaminophen will usually be the preferred drug for you. But if an NSAID is much more effective for controlling your pain, it is reasonable to use an NSAID, provided there are no problems with you taking an NSAID. Acetaminophen works as a painkiller; it has no effect on underlying arthritis. This means that if you are having a good day with little pain, you do not need to take any acetaminophen.

For rheumatoid arthritis and other inflammatory types of arthritis, NSAIDs are more effective than acetaminophen for controlling joint pain and swelling. Some people with rheumatoid arthritis or other types of inflammatory arthritis cannot take NSAIDs because of their side effects. For them, acetaminophen can help control pain.

ACETAMINOPHEN + NARCOTICS

(codeine/hydrocodone/oxycodone/propoxyphene)

Brand Names

Acetaminophen comes in combination with a range of different narcotic analgesics. Here are some of the common combinations and their brand names.

ACETAMINOPHEN + CODEINE: *Capital With Codeine, Phenaphen With Codeine, Tylenol With Codeine.*
ACETAMINOPHEN + HYDROCODONE: *Lortab, Lorcet, Lorcet Plus, Vicodin.*
ACETAMINOPHEN + OXYCODONE: *Percocet, Roxicet, Tylox.*
ACETAMINOPHEN + PROPOXYPHENE: *Darvocet N-50, Darvocet N-100.*

Drug Family

These are combination analgesics (painkillers) that combine a simple analgesic (acetaminophen) with a narcotic analgesic.

Families of Arthritis Problems Prescribed For

Acetaminophen + narcotic tablets are used for moderate to severe pain, whatever the cause. Analgesics that contain narcotics are usually prescribed only for pain that is not controlled by acetaminophen alone or an NSAID alone. Neither the acetaminophen component nor the narcotic component affects inflammation. Some studies have found that there is little difference in pain control between analgesic + narcotic combination tablets compared with acetaminophen alone or

NSAIDs alone. Many patients disagree and find acetaminophen + narcotic combinations useful for pain that is not controlled by an NSAID or by acetaminophen.

How It Works

No one knows for certain how acetaminophen works, but it may decrease the formation of chemicals called prostaglandins in the brain. Narcotics decrease pain by acting through specific narcotic receptors in the brain.

Avoid

Do not take these combination pills if you are allergic to acetaminophen or to the particular narcotic in the combination. Real allergic reactions are rare, but a lot of people get side effects such as nausea or feeling "spacy" from the narcotic component. Avoid analgesics that contain narcotics if you have had an addiction problem.

Take Precautions

- Do not drink alcohol while you are taking acetaminophen because it increases the risk of liver problems. Fasting may also increase the risk of liver damage. The maximum dose of acetaminophen that is safe in most people, a total dose of 4 g a day (equivalent to eight 500 mg tablets), may not be safe in people who are drinking alcohol or fasting. Talk to your physician if these apply to you.
- The maximum dose of acetaminophen that is safe in most adults, a total dose of 4 g a day (equivalent to eight 500 mg tablets), may not be safe in people who already have a liver problem. Talk to your physician if this applies to you.
- Acetaminophen in overdose can cause serious, and sometimes fatal, liver damage. Be careful that other prescription or over-the-counter medicines that contain aceta-

minophen do not push your total dose of acetaminophen up to an unsafe dose of more than 3 or 4 g a day.

- There is a small risk of becoming addicted to combination painkillers that contain narcotics. Take the tablets only for pain. If possible, limit the dose and how long you take them.

Side Effects

For the side effects of the acetaminophen part of the combination pill, look under ACETAMINOPHEN.

Side effects are caused by the narcotic component much more often than by acetaminophen. The side effects of narcotics taken in combination painkillers are usually mild. People vary in their sensitivity to different narcotics. Some people who cannot take preparations that contain codeine, for example, may be able to take other preparations containing hydrocodone, and vice versa.

Common: Nausea, vomiting, diarrhea, constipation, poor appetite, dizziness, light-headedness or feeling "spacy," and sleepiness are fairly common, but most people can find a preparation that they are able to take.

Less common: A real allergic reaction with rash, hives, or asthma is uncommon. Confusion, feeling very nervous or agitated, sleeping badly, feeling "high" and becoming addicted to the drug are uncommon but do occur.

Interactions with Other Drugs

Alcohol, barbiturates such as phenobarbitone (*Barbita*), isoniazid (*INH*): These drugs can increase the risk of liver damage from acetaminophen.

Warfarin (*Coumadin*): Acetaminophen, in a dose of more than 2 g a day, increases the anticoagulant (anti-blood clotting) effect of warfarin in some people. If you are taking warfarin to prevent blood clots and start taking acetaminophen regularly, you may need to have your blood monitored more frequently than usual, and your dose of warfarin may need to be changed.

Any other sedative drug: Narcotics make people sleepy, and an overdose can make people unconscious. Combining a narcotic with another sedative drug, such as alcohol, can be dangerous.

Important Information

- Don't take more than the prescribed dose.
- Many painkillers, both over-the-counter and prescription ones, contain acetaminophen. So if you are already taking acetaminophen, make sure that any additional painkillers you take do not push your total dose of acetaminophen up to more than 3 or 4 g a day.
- Don't drink alcohol while you are taking acetaminophen + narcotic combinations.
- Narcotics may cause drowsiness and affect your concentration while driving and performing other tasks.
- These painkillers contain a narcotic and can be addictive (read Comments).
- Acetaminophen and narcotics are dangerous in overdose. Keep these pills away from children.

Common Dose Sizes

ACETAMINOPHEN + CODEINE.

Tablet: *Tylenol #2,* Acetaminophen 300 mg with codeine 15 mg; *Tylenol #3,* Acetaminophen 300 mg with codeine 30 mg; *Tylenol #4,* Acetaminophen 300 mg with codeine 60 mg

ACETAMINOPHEN + HYDROCODONE.

Tablet: Hydrocodone 2.5 mg + acetaminophen 500 mg (*Lortab 2.5/500*); there are many other tablets with different doses of hydrocodone and acetaminophen. Some examples, with the mg hydrocodone/mg acetaminophen per tablet, are *Lortab 5/500; Lortab 7.5/500; Lorcet Plus* (*7.5/650*); *Lorcet 10/650; Vicodin* (*5/500*); *Vicodin ES* (*7.5/750*).

ACETAMINOPHEN + OXYCODONE.

Capsule: Acetaminophen 500 mg + oxycodone 5 mg (*Tylox*). Tablet: Acetaminophen 325 mg + oxycodone 5 mg (*Percocet, Roxicet*).

ACETAMINOPHEN + PROPOXYPHENE.

Tablet: Propoxyphene 50 mg + acetaminophen 325 mg (*Darvocet-N 50*); Propoxyphene 100 mg + acetaminophen 650 mg (*Darvocet-N 100*).

Usual Adult Doses

ACETAMINOPHEN + CODEINE:

The usual adult dose of most combination analgesic tablets is one to two tablets (that contain acetaminophen 300 mg + codeine 15 or 30 mg) up to every six to eight hours if needed.

ACETAMINOPHEN + HYDROCODONE:

The usual adult dose is 500 to 750 mg acetaminophen + 5 to 10 mg hydrocodone up to every six to eight hours if needed.

ACETAMINOPHEN + OXYCODONE:

The usual adult dose is one to two tablets (325 to 500 mg acetaminophen + 5 mg oxycodone) up to every six to eight hours if needed.

ACETAMINOPHEN + PROPOXYPHENE:

The usual adult dose is 50 to 100 mg propoxyphene + 325 to 650 mg acetaminophen up to every six to eight hours if needed.

Comments

There is some controversy about how narcotic analgesics should be used to control chronic "benign" pain, meaning chronic pain not caused by cancer. This is particularly true for the strong narcotics such as morphine, but to a lesser extent it is also true for the combination tablets that contain weak narcotics such as codeine and hydrocodone. Some physicians feel that the risk of addiction and abuse is too high and limit narcotic prescriptions to short periods, such as a few days, in all patients. Others are less rigid and believe that these analgesics can make life bearable for some people with chronic arthritis pain that cannot be controlled by other strategies. For example, I find them helpful to control pain at night in some people with severe osteoarthritis pain who cannot take NSAIDs because of their side effects. Most rheumatologists do not prescribe narcotics for fibromyalgia because they are not particularly helpful and because they can worsen the sleep disturbance.

Addiction to these painkillers is seldom a problem if they are taken to control pain. A clue to addictive behavior is if you are trying to get bigger doses of the drug and are not using the bigger doses to control pain. The risk of addiction is higher in people who themselves, or whose family members, have had an addiction problem (alcohol or drugs). I have a few rules for my patients about narcotic prescriptions.

1. Use the tablets only for pain, not to feel good.
2. If you don't have pain, don't take them.
3. Get all your narcotic prescriptions from one doctor and from one pharmacy.
4. Escalating the dose of your narcotic can be an early sign of a problem.
5. Never sell, swap, or hoard tablets.
6. If you are in the position of wanting to fool doctors or do illegal things such as forging signatures to get nar-

cotic prescriptions, then things are way out of control and you need to speak with your physician about getting help.

ACIPHEX (RABEPRAZOLE; SEE ***PROFILES OF COMMON PROTON PUMP INHIBITORS*** under OMEPRAZOLE)

ACTONEL (SEE RISEDRONATE)

ALENDRONATE

Brand Name

Fosamax.

Drug Family

Alendronate belongs to the family of drugs that prevent bone loss. It is a bisphosphonate.

Families of Arthritis Problems Prescribed For

Alendronate is used to treat and prevent osteoporosis. Remember that osteoporosis means "thin bones" and is not a type of arthritis. The aim of treating osteoporosis is to prevent fractures. Alendronate is also used to treat Paget's disease.

How It Works

Bone is continually replaced as it is absorbed, and then new bone is laid down to replace it. Alendronate slows down the resorption of bone but does not increase bone formation. Alendronate will usually stabilize your bone density or increase it slightly. In clinical trials, alendronate cuts the risk of fractures caused by osteoporosis by about half.

Avoid

Do not take alendronate if you are allergic to it, have poor kidney function, or have an esophagus (the food pipe that joins your mouth to your stomach) with a stricture or some other narrowing that causes food to get "hung up" when you swallow.

Take Precautions

If possible, avoid alendronate if you have a hiatal hernia or acid reflux (sometimes called GERD, or gastroesophageal reflux disease). Alendronate needs to be taken exactly as directed, otherwise it will not get into your bloodstream and will not work, or it may reflux up your esophagus and cause ulcers there.

Side Effects

Common: Mild gastrointestinal (GI) upset such as nausea, gas, constipation, and indigestion.

Rare: An allergic rash, difficulty swallowing, vomiting, and ulcers in the esophagus.

Interactions with Other Drugs

NSAIDs: GI side effects are more common when alendronate and NSAIDs are used together. However, many people with rheumatoid arthritis who take alendronate to treat or prevent osteoporosis caused by prednisone also take an NSAID for arthritis and tolerate the combination well.

Any drug: Alendronate is not absorbed into your body if you take it at the same time as any other drug or with food.

Important Information

- Alendronate should be taken with a full glass of water first thing in the morning.

• Do not eat or drink anything other than water for at least thirty minutes after taking alendronate. Even coffee or fruit juice will stop the alendronate from getting into your body. If you can wait an hour, so much the better, because more alendronate will be absorbed into your body.

• After you have taken alendronate, stay upright. This is so that the tablet doesn't reflux back up your esophagus.

• Take alendronate by itself. Delay taking your other medicines for at least an hour.

Common Dose Sizes

Tablet: 10 mg, 70 mg.

Usual Adult Doses

The usual dose of alendronate for osteoporosis is 10 mg a day or 70 mg once a week. The once-a-week dose is more convenient, causes less GI side effects, and is as effective as the daily dose. Alendronate stabilizes osteoporosis but does not cure it, so treatment needs to continue for a long time.

For Paget's disease, the usual dose of alendronate is 40 mg a day for six months. This often controls Paget's disease, but another course of treatment may be needed.

Comments

Osteoporosis is a common problem, particularly in women after menopause and in people taking corticosteroids. Osteoporosis is diagnosed by measuring your bone density, often with a type of scan known as DEXA (dual-energy X-ray absorptiometry). The usual program to treat or prevent osteoporosis also includes stopping smoking and alcohol, increasing exercise, and taking calcium supplements and a low dose of vitamin D, often as part of a multivitamin tablet.

Alendronate is the bisphosphonate that has the most supporting evidence showing that it actually decreases the risk of fractures. Don't forget that the aim of treating osteoporosis is to prevent fractures and that many fractures are caused by falls. Simple things can reduce your risk of falling. Some of these may apply to you. Get rid of loose throw rugs and other objects that can trip you, have nonslip surfaces, use a cane if you need one, don't hurry—that telephone can keep ringing—and keep a night-light on so that you can see your way to the bathroom. People with poor vision are more likely to fall, so have your vision checked from time to time. Alcohol and medicines that affect your balance, such as many kinds of sleeping pills, increase your risk of falling. Avoid them if possible.

ALLOPURINOL

Brand Names

Lopurin, Zyloprim.

Drug Family

Allopurinol belongs to the family of drugs that prevent attacks of gout by decreasing the uric acid level in your blood. Allopurinol is sometimes classified as a xanthine oxidase inhibitor because it works by blocking the enzyme xanthine oxidase.

Families of Arthritis Problems Prescribed For

Allopurinol is used to *prevent* gout. It is particularly useful for people who have kidney stones caused by uric acid or who have tophi. Tophi are lumps of uric acid that can be deposited in different parts of your body, most often on the elbows or ears.

How It Works

Allopurinol decreases the uric acid levels in your blood by decreasing the amount of uric acid your body makes. It does this by blocking an enzyme called xanthine oxidase.

Avoid

Do not take allopurinol if you are allergic to it.

Take Precautions

- The dose of allopurinol often needs to be lower in older people, in people taking diuretics ("water pills"), and in people with decreased kidney function.
- If you are also taking azathioprine (*Imuran*) or mercaptopurine (*Purinethol*), types of anticancer drugs that are sometimes used for arthritis-related problems, the dose of these drugs will need to be decreased a lot (see Interactions with Other Drugs).
- Blood tests are usually taken from time to time to check your blood count, liver function, and kidney function, particularly soon after you start treatment. If your blood uric-acid level is high, the drop in the uric acid in response to treatment can be a useful guide to the dose of allopurinol you need.

Side Effects

Common: Starting allopurinol can sometimes bring on an attack of gout. So if you have recently had an attack of gout, most physicians wait until it has been controlled with an NSAID or colchicine before starting you on treatment with allopurinol.

A mild allergic rash is fairly common, particularly in the first few weeks of treatment. If this happens, stop the allopurinol and contact your doctor. If the problem is mild and is limited to a slight rash, it may be possible, once the rash has cleared, for your physician to restart the allopurinol and see how you do.

Rare: There is a serious but very rare allergic reaction to allopurinol called the "allopurinol hypersensitivity syndrome." People with this side effect have a severe rash, often with blisters and peeling skin, and also have kidney and liver problems. The risk is higher in people who already have poor kidney function and in people who are also taking diuretics ("water pills").

Allopurinol can rarely damage the bone marrow so that there is decreased production of the different components of blood (white blood cells, red blood cells, and platelets).

Interactions with Other Drugs

Azathioprine (*Imuran*) and mercaptopurine (*Purinethol*): Allopurinol slows the breakdown of these anticancer drugs, and this means that, unless far smaller doses than usual of azathioprine or mercaptopurine are prescribed, there will be serious bone-marrow problems. Most physicians try to avoid the combination of allopurinol and either of these drugs. But sometimes, particularly in people who get gout after they have had an organ transplant, the choices are limited and they are used together. If allopurinol is prescribed with azathioprine or mercaptopurine, their doses have to be decreased a lot and very careful monitoring of the blood count is needed.

Warfarin (*Coumadin*): Allopurinol can increase the anticoagulant (anti-blood clotting) effect of warfarin in some people. If you are taking warfarin to prevent blood clots and start taking allopurinol, you may need to have your blood monitored more frequently than usual, and your dose of warfarin may need to be changed.

Cyclophosphamide (*Cytoxan*): The sensitivity of your bone marrow to cyclophosphamide can be increased when allopurinol and cyclophosphamide are combined.

Ampicillin (*Omnipen* and many other brand names) and Amoxicillin (*Amoxil* and many other brand names): These antibiotics can increase the risk of an allergic rash, usually mild, with allopurinol.

Thiazide diuretics (many brand and generic preparations): Diuretics increase the risk of allopurinol hypersensitivity. We are not sure how. Most diuretics also increase the uric acid level in your blood, and in people with gout, physicians usually try to use alternative drugs—say, for treating high blood pressure. However, many people with gout also need diuretics for a problem such as heart failure, and it is often not possible to avoid using diuretics and allopurinol together.

Theophylline (*Theo-Dur* and many other brand names): Allopurinol can increase blood levels of theophylline; the dose of theophylline may need to be decreased.

Important Information

• Allopurinol is taken regularly to prevent gout. Your risk for getting gout does not usually go away. So to keep attacks of gout away, allopurinol often needs to be taken for many years, or indefinitely. Allopurinol may not completely prevent attacks of acute gout. If you have an attack of gout while you are taking allopurinol, remember that allopurinol has no effect on the pain and swelling of the acute attack. A common mistake people make is to take their allopurinol only when they get an attack of gout.

• If you develop a rash while you are taking allopurinol, stop the drug and contact your doctor.

• If you have tophi that you can see or feel, they may get smaller with allopurinol treatment. This happens very slowly, often over months or years.

Common Dose Sizes

Tablets: 100 mg and 300 mg.

Usual Adult Doses

The usual adult starting dose of allopurinol is 100 mg or 200 mg once a day. The dose can be increased every couple of weeks, if needed, depending on how your blood uric acid level responds. In older people, lower starting doses such as 50 mg or 100 mg a day, are sometimes used. Most people end up taking about 200 mg or 300 mg a day, but some people with a very high uric acid level may need bigger doses, sometimes up to 600 mg a day.

People with poor kidney function should take lower doses of allopurinol. The worse the kidney function, the lower the dose of allopurinol needed.

Comments

Most rheumatologists wait until someone has had at least two attacks of gout before starting treatment with a drug such as allopurinol to drop the uric acid level. This is because some people have very few attacks of gout spread over their lifetime. These people may not need treatment with a medicine that they have to take every day, perhaps forever, to prevent something that may happen only once or twice in a lifetime.

When someone starts allopurinol for the first time, most rheumatologists also prescribe an NSAID, or a drug called colchicine, for a few months. This is to control any acute attacks of gout that may be brought on by starting allopurinol.

Remember, allopurinol is preventive treatment. It needs to be taken regularly. If you stop taking allopurinol, your blood uric acid level goes back to where it started within a few weeks. Allopurinol has no anti-inflammatory activity and does not help an acute attack of gout.

A high uric acid level is common in healthy people and does not mean that they have gout. A high uric acid level by itself, without attacks of gout, almost never needs treatment with a drug such as allopurinol, but it can be an indicator that lifestyle changes may be in order—for example, losing weight or drinking less alcohol.

AMBIEN (SEE ZOLPIDEM)

AMITRIPTYLINE

Brand Names

Elavil, Endep, and *Enovil.*

Drug Family

Amitriptyline is an antidepressant. But for people with arthritis problems, it is often used for other effects, such as improving sleep and decreasing pain. Amitriptyline, like most of the older antidepressants, belongs to the tricyclic antidepressant family. There are many different types of antidepressants with different side effect profiles. These are summarized in the table *Profiles of Common Antidepressant Drugs,* which follows on page 37.

Families of Arthritis Problems Prescribed For

For people with arthritis problems, amitriptyline is used most often to treat fibromyalgia, but it is also used to improve sleep and to help control pain, particularly pain caused by nerve damage.

How It Works

Amitriptyline and many other antidepressants work by increasing the amount of chemicals that act as messengers in the nerve junctions. Amitriptyline increases the concentrations of chemicals called norepinephrine and serotonin in the nerve junctions.

Avoid

Do not take amitriptyline if you are allergic to it. Minor side effects are fairly common, but a real allergic reaction is rare. People who have side effects with one antidepressant may be able to take another with a slightly different side effect profile. Do not take tricyclic antidepressants such as amitriptyline if you are taking or have recently taken a monoamine oxidase inhibitor antidepressant (see Interactions with Other Drugs). Amitriptyline is avoided soon after a heart attack and in people who have certain types of heart-rhythm problems.

Take Precautions

- Amitriptyline may cause you to be sleepy and may affect your ability to drive or operate machinery.
- Men who have prostate trouble may find that it becomes more difficult to pass urine.
- Dry eyes and dry mouth, which are problems in Sjogren's syndrome, can get worse.
- Amitriptyline can bring on glaucoma (high pressure in the eyeball), particularly in people who are predisposed to it.

Side Effects

Common: Sleepiness is common, and because of this, amitriptyline is often used to improve sleep. Sometimes people still feel "hung-over" the next day. Amitriptyline can cause your mouth and eyes to feel dry, can blur vision slightly, and cause constipation and, particularly in men with prostate problems, some difficulty passing urine. These side effects are called "anticholinergic" side effects, and they vary between antidepressants. You may find that your body gets used to some of these side effects and that you notice them less as you take amitriptyline for a longer time.

Less common: Most people get sleepy when they take amitriptyline, but some people find the opposite. Dizziness when standing up suddenly, tremor (shakiness), nausea, weight gain, confusion, and stomach upset can occur.

Rare: Rare side effects are bone marrow problems, liver problems, seizures, hair loss, and heart-rhythm problems.

Interactions with Other Drugs

Alcohol and other sedatives: These increase the sedative effects of amitriptyline.

Cimetidine (*Tagamet*): Cimetidine slows the breakdown of amitriptyline in your body, and you may need a slightly lower dose of amitriptyline.

Monoamine oxidase inhibitor antidepressants—isocarboxazid (*Marplan*), phenelzine (*Nardil*), and tranylcypromine (*Parnate*): There is an increased risk of serious heart and blood-pressure side effects, and even death, if these drugs are taken at the same time or within a few weeks of taking tricyclic antidepressants such as amitriptyline.

Guanethidine (*Ismelin*), guanadrel (*Hylorel*), and clonidine (*Catapres*): Amitriptyline can block the blood-pressure-lowering effects of these antihypertensive drugs.

Warfarin (*Coumadin*): Amitriptyline can increase the anticoagulant (anti-blood clotting) effect of warfarin in some people. If you are taking warfarin to prevent blood clots and start taking amitriptyline, you may need to have your blood monitored more frequently than usual, and your dose of warfarin may need to be changed.

Tramadol (*Ultram*): Amitriptyline and other antidepressants can increase the risk of seizures with tramadol.

Cisapride (*Propulsid*): Amitriptyline and many other antidepressants may increase the risk of an abnormal heart rhythm with cisapride.

Important Information

- Start with a low dose of amitriptyline and build up slowly.
- Avoid alcohol while you are taking amitriptyline.
- Amitriptyline is dangerous in overdose. Keep it away from children.
- If you are taking amitriptyline to treat depression, it is important to remember that the antidepressant effects can be delayed for several weeks.
- If you are taking amitriptyline to improve sleep, take it a few hours before bedtime because it does not work fast.

Common Dose Sizes

Tablets: 10 mg, 25 mg, 50 mg, and bigger sizes.

Usual Adult Doses

The starting dose of amitriptyline for fibromyalgia, often 10 mg, taken two hours before bedtime, is lower than the dose prescribed for other problems such as depression. Most people with fibromyalgia take 50 mg or less of amitriptyline at night. The dose used to treat depression is higher, usually in the range of 75 mg to 150 mg a day.

Comments

The side effects of amitriptyline tend to be more noticeable soon after you start it. That is one of the reasons why, in people with fibromyalgia, I usually start with a very low dose of 10 mg a day. This dose can then be increased slowly to find an individual dose that improves your sleep and does not cause side effects. The benefits of drugs such as amitriptyline for fibromyalgia are, on average, modest. It can help with some of the symptoms of fibromyalgia, probably by improving the quality of sleep, but it usually does not make the symptoms disappear.

There are many antidepressants available. They have different chemical structures and work in slightly different ways. The older tricyclics block the uptake of the chemical transmitters, norepinephrine and serotonin, back into the nerve, and by doing this they increase the concentrations of these chemicals in the nerve terminals. The newer antidepressants are more selective for a chemical, serotonin, and are often called selective serotonin reuptake inhibitors (SSRIs). The individual antidepressant drugs, as treatment for depression, are on average equally effective. But as happens with all drugs, different people respond better to a particular drug. The various drugs do have different side effect profiles, particularly regarding sedative effects (drowsiness), anticholinergic effects (dry eyes, dry mouth, trouble passing urine) and GI symptoms (usually nausea). These are shown

PROFILES OF COMMON ANTIDEPRESSANT DRUGS

Generic name	*Brand name*	*Anticholinergic*	*Drowsiness*	*GI symptoms*
FIRST-GENERATION ANTIDEPRESSANTS				
TRICYCLICS				
Amitriptyline	*Elavil*	++++	++++	0/+
Doxepin	*Sinequan*	++++	++++	0/+
Imipramine	*Tofranil*	+++	+++	+
Nortriptyline	*Pamelor*	++	+	0/+
SECOND-GENERATION ANTIDEPRESSANTS				
Maprotiline	*Ludiomil*	++	+++	0/+
Trazodone	*Desyrel*	0	++++	+
Bupropion	*Wellbutrin*	0	0	+
THIRD-GENERATION ANTIDEPRESSANTS				
SELECTIVE SEROTONIN REUPTAKE INHIBITORS (SSRIs)				
Fluoxetine	*Prozac*	0	0	+++
Paroxetine	*Paxil*	0/+	0/+	+++
Sertraline	*Zoloft*	0	0	+++
NOREPINEPHRINE/SEROTONIN REUPTAKE INHIBITORS				
Venlafaxine	*Effexor*	+	+	+++

The monoamine oxidase inhibitor antidepressants are not included in the table. They can have very dangerous side effects and interactions with other drugs. It is best that they are prescribed and monitored by a psychiatrist.

in the table on page 37. Sexual problems and fatigue may be more common with the SSRIs than with the older antidepressants.

ANAPROX (SEE NAPROXEN)

ANSAID (SEE FLURBIPROFEN)

ARAVA (SEE LEFLUNOMIDE)

AREDIA (SEE PAMIDRONATE)

ARTHROTEC (SEE DICLOFENAC)

ARTIFICIAL TEARS

Brand Names

There are many artificial tear preparations available. Here are some: *Artificial Tears, Bion Tears, Cellufresh, Hypotears, Isopto Alkaline, Isopto Plain, Isopto Tears, Just Tears, Nature's Tears, Ocucoat, Ocucoat PF, Refresh, Refresh Plus, Tears Naturelle, Tears Naturelle II, Tears Naturelle Free,* and *Ultra Tears.*

Drug Family

These drops or ointments protect the eyes against dryness. Many contain hydroxypropyl methyl cellulose or a similar chemical that holds onto liquid and keeps your eyes moist.

Families of Arthritis Problems Prescribed For

Artificial tears are used to treat dry eyes, which are often part of Sjogren's syndrome.

How It Works

Artificial tears keep your eyes moist by providing a lubricant, and they also thicken your tears.

Take Precautions

- If your eyes become irritated with some preparations, this may be caused by a preservative. Use a preservative-free preparation if this happens.
- Do not use these drops with contact lenses unless they are designed for use with contact lenses.

Side Effects

Common: Mild blurring of vision.

Less common: Irritation of the eye that may be caused by a preservative agent.

Important Information

- It is much more effective to use the drops regularly, even when your eyes do not feel dry, rather than to wait until your eyes feel dry.

Usual Adult Doses

The usual dose is one drop every four to eight hours, but this varies a lot. People with very dry eyes may need to put drops in every couple of hours.

Comments

Lubricant eye ointments can be used at night. Their effect lasts longer than the liquid drops, but they blur vision more, so most people prefer not to use them during the day. Don't forget other tricks for keeping your eyes moist, such as wearing glasses with side shields and avoiding direct wind and rooms that are over–air conditioned.

ASCRIPTIN (SEE CHOLINE SALICYLATE)

ASPIRIN

Brand Names

Anacin, Ascriptin, A.S.A, Bayer Aspirin, Bufferin, Easprin, Ecotrin, Zorprin.

Sometimes Called

Aspirin is sometimes abbreviated to ASA, which is short for acetylsalicylic acid.

Drug Family

Aspirin belongs to the nonsteroidal anti-inflammatory drug (NSAID) family. There are two big groups of NSAIDs, divided by whether they inhibit both cyclo-oxygenase (COX) enzymes, COX-1 and COX-2, or are more selective for COX-2. Aspirin inhibits both COX-1 and COX-2.

Families of Arthritis Problems Prescribed For

Aspirin is used for three major reasons.

1. To treat pain and inflammation—analgesic and anti-inflammatory effects. Aspirin is used for all kinds of painful problems, whether they affect the joints or not. Aspirin is also used to treat many kinds of arthritis problems, such as rheumatoid arthritis (RA), osteoarthritis (OA), rheumatic fever, Still's disease (also known as juvenile rheumatoid arthritis, or JRA), Kawasaki disease, and bursitis. NSAIDs decrease pain and inflammation, but they do not change the progression of arthritis.

2. To treat fever—antipyretic effects. Aspirin brings down a temperature caused by infection or inflammation.
3. To prevent blood clots—antithrombotic effects. Aspirin is famous because this simple drug, if it is given to someone who is having a heart attack, cuts the risk of death in half. Aspirin makes the platelets in your blood less sticky. This makes it less likely that the clots that can start a heart attack will form. Aspirin is used to treat and prevent heart attacks and strokes in many people, with or without arthritis problems. Aspirin is also sometimes used to prevent a stroke or a heart attack in people with systemic lupus erythematosus (SLE) or with a problem called the anticardiolipin antibody syndrome.

How It Works

Aspirin inhibits the enzymes COX-1 and COX-2. Inhibiting these cyclo-oxygenase enzymes decreases the formation of chemicals called prostaglandins. Decreasing the prostaglandins made by COX-2 is anti-inflammatory, which is usually why we use NSAIDs. Most NSAIDs inhibit both COX-1 and COX-2. Inhibiting COX-1 makes platelets in your blood less sticky. Aspirin has very long-lasting effects on platelets, and that is why it is used to prevent heart attacks and strokes. COX-1 also protects the stomach from ulcers, and blocking COX-1 may be why the risk of peptic ulcers is increased with aspirin and many other NSAIDs.

Avoid

Do not take aspirin if you are allergic to it. People who have had a serious allergic reaction (swelling of the face and tongue, and wheezing) to one NSAID can have the same reaction with others. People with asthma or nasal polyps are more likely to be allergic to NSAIDs.

Aspirin is generally avoided in children and if someone has an active peptic ulcer, is bleeding, or is pregnant.

Take Precautions

• NSAIDs can cause fluid retention and can worsen heart failure and high blood pressure.

• Some people have a higher risk for getting peptic ulcers caused by NSAIDs. Risk factors are being older than 65 years, having had a previous peptic ulcer, having had a previous bleeding ulcer, and taking a corticosteroid. In people who are at higher risk for peptic ulcers caused by NSAIDs, most rheumatologists would avoid an NSAID, if possible. If this is not possible, then prescribing misoprostol (see MISOPROSTOL—*Cytotec*) or a proton pump inhibitor (see OMEPRAZOLE—*Prilosec*) to protect against peptic ulcers caused by NSAIDs is an option. Another option is to use a COX-2 selective NSAID (see CELECOXIB—*Celebrex* and ROFECOXIB—*Vioxx*). None of these choices is foolproof, and peptic ulcers can still happen.

• NSAIDs have to be used carefully in people who have asthma, a bleeding problem, or liver or kidney problems.

• If you are taking NSAIDs regularly, blood tests will be done from time to time to check your blood count (in case you are losing blood slowly from an ulcer that you may not know about), your creatinine (for kidney function), and liver enzymes. People who take diuretics ("water pills") or ACE (angiotensin converting enzyme) inhibitors—a family of drugs that lowers blood pressure—people with diabetes, heart failure, or existing kidney problems are more likely to have kidney problems caused by NSAIDs. These people may need more frequent blood tests to check their kidney function.

Side Effects

Common: NSAIDs are one of the most common medicines we take. Many people tolerate NSAIDs reasonably well. GI problems, usually indigestion or heartburn, are the most common reasons people stop NSAIDs. One of the less common but more severe side effects is a serious peptic ulcer problem. NSAIDs often cause some fluid retention with a little ankle swelling.

Less common: Peptic ulcers can be silent, without warning symptoms such as indigestion. Small ulcers occur in many people taking NSAIDs without their even knowing it. In people at higher risk (older than 65 years, a previous peptic ulcer, a previous bleeding ulcer, and combined treatment with a corticosteroid), the annual risk of a serious ulcer problem with nonselective NSAIDs can be as high as three out of every 100 people.

Blood pressure can increase in some people, usually by a small amount. Abnormal liver function tests (usually mild), rashes, ringing in the ears, and a feeling of lightheadedness or feeling "spacy" can occur.

Rare: Bleeding from an ulcer, perforation of the bowel, liver problems, and kidney problems can occur. People who are allergic to aspirin and who have wheezing, a lumpy and itchy rash, and swelling of the tongue or face when they take aspirin are often allergic to other NSAIDs. Reye's syndrome is a very rare problem that caused liver failure and coma in children treated with aspirin for a viral illness. It virtually disappeared after the recommendation that aspirin should not be used in children.

Interactions with Other Drugs

Antacids: Antacids can decrease the effect of aspirin by increasing its excretion in urine.

Warfarin (*Coumadin*): Aspirin can increase the anticoagulant (anti-blood clotting) effect of warfarin in some people. If you are taking warfarin to prevent blood clots and start taking aspirin, you may need to have your blood monitored more frequently than usual, and your dose of warfarin may need to be changed. If possible, NSAIDs such as aspirin are avoided in people taking warfarin or other anticoagulants because the effects of aspirin on platelets increase the risk of bleeding.

NSAIDs: A combination of two NSAIDs is avoided because it does not improve the control of inflammation but does increase the risk of side effects. But if someone on an NSAID needs aspirin to prevent a heart attack or stroke, then a low dose of aspirin is often prescribed with the other NSAID.

Methotrexate (*Rheumatrex*): Aspirin and other NSAIDs can increase the concentrations of methotrexate in your blood, usually only by a small amount. In rheumatology practice, with the low doses of methotrexate used, this interaction is seldom important, and methotrexate is often prescribed for rheumatoid arthritis, together with an NSAID.

Lithium: Many NSAIDs can increase lithium levels. Lithium levels are usually monitored, and the dose of lithium can be decreased if needed.

Diuretics ("water pills") or ACE (angiotensin converting enzyme) inhibitors—a family of drugs that lowers blood pressure: Many NSAIDs blunt the ability of these drugs to lower blood pressure.

Important Information

- Taking NSAIDs with food is a good idea and may protect you from indigestion, but it does not prevent peptic ulcers.
- The effects of aspirin on platelet stickiness are long lasting. To prevent minor bleeding, you may be asked to stop aspirin a week or two before some types of surgery.

• One of the signs that you may be bleeding from the stomach is if you have pitch-black bowel movements. Bowel movements with altered blood, in addition to being black, are also often runny and very smelly. If this happens, contact your doctor immediately.

Common Dose Sizes

Tablets: 81 mg, 325 mg, 500 mg; Tablets, enteric-coated: 165 mg, 325 mg, 500 mg; Tablets, timed or controlled-release (slow-release): 800 mg.

Usual Adult Doses

The usual adult dose of aspirin to decrease fever or to treat minor pain is one or two 325 mg aspirin tablets taken every six hours. Higher doses, for example, up to 4 g a day (equivalent to a total of twelve of the 325 mg tablets a day), can be used to treat inflammation. Very low doses of aspirin, 81 mg to 325 mg a day, are used to prevent blood clotting.

Comments

To prevent heart attacks or strokes, aspirin has an advantage over all the other NSAIDs because it is the only one that has long-lasting effects on platelet stickiness. Coated aspirin or delayed-release aspirin may cause less indigestion than regular aspirin but can still cause peptic ulcers.

Most people take NSAIDs for arthritis pain. There is no convincing evidence that one NSAID is more effective than another for arthritis pain. But people respond differently, and you may find that a particular NSAID suits you best. There are many NSAIDs on the market. I don't think there is much point in trying a lot of different NSAIDs to get greater effect. If two or three don't help much, it usually means that some other type of treatment may be better for you.

Some people with osteoarthritis find that NSAIDs and acetaminophen reduce their pain by about the same amount. If this is the case for you, take acetaminophen, because it is safer. Rheumatoid arthritis causes a lot more inflammation than osteoarthritis, and NSAIDs usually control the symptoms of RA better than acetaminophen does. People vary a lot. Some people with RA tell me they find that NSAIDs make very little difference to their symptom control. For them, the risks outweigh the benefits, and I suggest that they do not take an NSAID. Other people with RA find that NSAIDs help them a lot. RA is virtually never controlled by an NSAID alone, so a disease-modifying antirheumatic drug (DMARD) is introduced early in the treatment plan.

There are many unanswered questions about NSAIDs. Do the serious ulcer problems caused by older NSAIDs in relatively few people mean that everyone should be treated with a new COX-2 selective NSAID—although it may cost more? Are there side effects from the new COX-2 selective NSAIDs that we don't know about yet? In people at higher risk for ulcers, are COX-2 selective NSAIDs safer than a nonselective NSAID taken with a stomach protective agent? We don't know the answers to these questions. My approach is not to change people who are stable on their older NSAID to a newer COX-2 selective drug. In people at higher risk for NSAID ulcer problems, I discuss the choices available and use a COX-2 selective drug or an older NSAID with either misoprostol (see MISOPROSTOL—*Cytotec*) or a proton pump inhibitor (see OMEPRAZOLE—*Prilosec*) to protect against ulcers. As more information becomes available, we will have clearer answers to these questions. I suspect that COX-2 selective NSAIDs, because they are equally effective and are likely to be safer, will replace the nonselective NSAIDs as the first choice for most people with arthritis who need NSAIDs.

AURANOFIN

Brand Names
Ridaura.

Sometimes Called
Oral gold.

Drug Family
Auranofin is a disease-modifying antirheumatic drug (DMARD).

Families of Arthritis Problems Prescribed For
Auranofin is most often used as a DMARD for rheumatoid arthritis. It is also sometimes used to treat psoriatic arthritis.

How It Works
We are not sure how gold works in rheumatoid arthritis. Gold affects some of the white blood cell functions, but it does not suppress your immune system and so does not increase your risk of infection.

Avoid
Avoid gold if you are allergic to it, if you have had serious bone marrow problems, or if your kidney function is poor. Gold is avoided in pregnancy.

Take Precautions

- Gold can cause, and worsen, dermatitis or eczema. If you develop a skin rash, stop the drug and contact your doctor.
- Gold has to be used cautiously in people with decreased liver or kidney function.

• Your blood count and urine will be tested regularly. These tests are usually done fairly frequently, perhaps every couple of weeks, after you start gold. After a while they will be done once a month and then, once you have been stable on treatment for a while, less often. The white cell count and platelet count in your blood will be checked, and if they drop significantly, gold may need to be stopped. Your urine will be checked for protein and, if you start to show protein in the urine, gold may need to be stopped.

• Avoid spending time in the sun, because gold can increase your skin's sensitivity to sunlight.

Side Effects

Common: Stomach problems such as loose bowel movements, diarrhea, gas, and cramping are common, and although they are not serious, some people cannot take auranofin because of these side effects. Itching, skin rash, mouth ulcers, and protein in the urine are also fairly common.

Rare: Much less common but more serious are a severe skin rash with skin peeling, other serious allergic reactions, serious bone-marrow problems with a low white cell count or low platelet count, liver problems, peripheral nerve problems, fever, and lung problems.

Interactions with Other Drugs

Other DMARDs (penicillamine, hydroxychloroquine, immunosuppressants): The risk of side effects with other DMARDs may be increased if they are used in combination with gold. Having said this, DMARDs are often used in combination to try and improve the control of RA.

Important Information

• Monitoring is important. Don't skip your lab checkups.

• Gold works slowly, but if you have had no response after six months of treatment, it is time to think about another DMARD.

• If you develop a skin rash, stop the gold and contact your doctor.

Common Dose Sizes

Capsule: 3 mg.

Usual Adult Doses

The usual adult dose of auranofin is 6 mg a day. If, after a few months, your response to this dose is not good, and if you have had no side effects, a dose of 9 mg a day can be tried.

Comments

Auranofin is a relatively weak DMARD. I sometimes use it for people with RA that is mild or early, and some of them do very well. The combination of auranofin with methotrexate has been tested and, on average, was no more effective than methotrexate alone. Side effects were more common with the combination treatment. As far as the choice between oral gold and gold injection goes, I think that oral gold is probably less effective than gold injections, but oral gold also causes side effects less often. Auranofin suits some people very well, but the frequency of side effects, most often nuisance side effects, means that a lot of people can't take it.

AZATHIOPRINE

Brand Name

Imuran.

Drug Family

Azathioprine is an anticancer drug that modulates the immune system. It was first used to treat cancer and was then found to be useful for treating some rheumatic problems. Much smaller doses are used to treat rheumatic problems than are used to treat cancer. Side effects are much less common with these lower doses than with cancer chemotherapy doses.

Families of Arthritis Problems Prescribed For

Azathioprine is used to treat rheumatoid arthritis, particularly in people who cannot take other DMARDs, such as methotrexate. It is also used to treat systemic lupus erythematosus, dermatomyositis or polymyositis, and other connective tissue problems. Azathioprine is sometimes used as "maintenance" treatment in people with vasculitis to hold the problem in remission. In people who need high doses of corticosteroids to control their autoimmune problem, azathioprine acts as a "steroid-sparing" agent, and the dose of corticosteroid can be decreased.

How It Works

Azathioprine interferes with DNA synthesis, particularly in cells that regulate your immune response. Azathioprine, in the doses used in rheumatology, does not usually change your blood counts much. So azathioprine is not working by killing off a lot of your blood cells. Rather, it selectively affects those cells that are driving the immune response and causing the problem.

Avoid

Do not take azathioprine if you are allergic to it. Azathioprine has a serious drug interaction with allopurinol, and this combination is usually avoided. Azathioprine is avoided in pregnancy, if possible.

Take Precautions

• Caution is needed in people with decreased liver or kidney function.

• Your blood count will be checked from time to time, often every one to two weeks initially, and then less often once you are on a stable dose of azathioprine. Liver function tests are also checked, but much less often.

• Because azathioprine suppresses your immune system, you should take seriously any infections that you may get and have them treated early.

Side Effects

Common: GI symptoms such as vomiting, diarrhea, and nausea are common but not serious. About 25 percent of people find they cannot take azathioprine because of these side effects. Mild changes in liver enzyme tests are common, but serious liver problems are rare.

Less common: Azathioprine can suppress your bone marrow and cause a low white blood cell count or a low platelet count. How much azathioprine affects your bone marrow depends on the dose you take and how sensitive you are to it. If your blood count is monitored regularly, bone marrow suppression is not usually a problem. There is a particular gene found in one in 300 people that makes them very sensitive to azathioprine. Testing for this gene will probably become available soon.

Mouth ulcers, rash, and an increased risk of infection are seen. Infections can be regular infections such as pneumonia, but can also be less common infections such as tuberculosis. Shingles (also called herpes zoster), a painful blistering rash caused by reactivation of the chicken pox virus, is more common in people taking azathioprine.

Rare: Pancreatitis, serious liver problems, serious lung problems, and serious allergic reactions are rare. Azathioprine may slightly increase the risk of some malignancies, such as lymphoma and leukemia, but the studies are conflicting and some show no increased risk of cancer.

Interactions with Other Drugs

Allopurinol (*Zyloprim*): Azathioprine (*Imuran*) and mercaptopurine (*Purinethol*) interact with allopurinol. Allopurinol slows the breakdown of these drugs, and this means that unless far smaller doses than usual of azathioprine or mercaptopurine are prescribed, there will be serious bone marrow problems. Most physicians try to avoid the combination of allopurinol and either of these drugs. But sometimes, particularly in people who get gout after they have had an organ transplant, the choices are limited and they are used together. If allopurinol is prescribed with azathioprine or mercaptopurine, their dose has to be decreased a lot, and very careful monitoring of the blood count is needed.

Other immunosuppressants: All drugs that suppress the immune system increase the risk of side effects such as infection. The more the immune system is suppressed, the higher the risk. High doses of corticosteroids, alone or with other drugs such as azathioprine, increase the risk of infection.

Live vaccines: Some vaccines are given as a weaker strain of a live virus. These vaccines are usually avoided in people taking drugs such as azathioprine, which can suppress the immune system.

Important Information

- Avoid becoming pregnant while you are taking azathioprine.
- Do not take more than the prescribed dose.
- Regular monitoring of your blood count is important.
- Avoid immunizations, except for influenza and pneumonia, unless approved by your physician.

• Contact your doctor if you develop any serious or prolonged infection or fever.

Common Dose Sizes

Tablet: 50 mg.

Usual Adult Doses

Azathioprine is usually dosed according to your body weight. The usual dose is in the range of 1 to 2 mg per kg per day. So for a 75 kg adult (about 165 lbs), the dose would usually be between 75 mg and 150 mg a day.

Comments

Azathioprine is often not as effective as some of the other DMARDs for RA, but it is useful for some people who cannot take other DMARDs. The response to azathioprine in RA comes on slowly, often taking two to three months. Azathioprine in combination with methotrexate has been tested in RA and, on average, this combination is no better than methotrexate alone. Azathioprine is not as effective as cyclophosphamide for treating severe kidney problems caused by lupus. But azathioprine is very useful for many less serious types of SLE, including some types of kidney problems. In many other autoimmune problems, azathioprine, often in combination with a corticosteroid, helps to control the problem.

Most people who stop azathioprine do so not because of serious side effects that threaten their life or health but because of uncomfortable GI symptoms. These problems can sometimes be improved by splitting the dose so that smaller doses are taken twice a day rather than a bigger dose once a day. In people who do not get GI symptoms, azathioprine is usually well tolerated.

AZULFIDINE (SEE SULFASALAZINE)

BENEMID (SEE PROBENECID)

BUTAZOLIDIN (SEE PHENYLBUTAZONE)

CALCITONIN

Brand Names
Cibacalcin (human), *Miacalcin* (salmon).

Sometimes Called
Salmon calcitonin, Human calcitonin.

Drug Family
Calcitonin falls into the family of drugs that prevents bone loss.

Families of Arthritis Problems Prescribed For
Injectable calcitonin is used to treat and prevent osteoporosis and to treat Paget's disease. Calcitonin nasal spray is used to treat and prevent osteoporosis.

How It Works
Calcitonin is a hormone that slows the breakdown of bone.

Avoid
Do not take calcitonin if you are allergic to it.

Take Precautions

• Most physicians do a skin test with a low dose of the calcitonin injection to see if you are allergic to it. Allergy to nasal calcitonin is rare, and usually no special precautions are taken with it.

• In people with osteoporosis, bone density is often measured every few years to guide treatment. Blood tests, such as the concentration of an enzyme called alkaline phosphatase, or markers of bone turnover measured in your urine, can help guide treatment in Paget's disease.

Side Effects

Common: Calcitonin injections can cause flushing, headache, nausea, diarrhea, and redness at the injection site. Nasal calcitonin is much less likely to cause side effects, but it can cause nasal irritation.

Less common: Allergy and rash are less common, particularly with nasal calcitonin. A drop in the blood level of calcium is rare.

Important Information

• With the calcitonin nasal spray, use alternate nostrils to minimize irritation to your nose.

• Most calcitonin preparations are stable at room temperature for a couple of weeks, but it is best to store them in the refrigerator (not the freezer). Read the instructions that come with your preparation.

Common Dose Sizes

Salmon calcitonin injection: 200 units/ml (2 ml), 100 units/ml (1 ml); Nasal spray: 2 ml bottle with 200 International Units (IU) per spray; Human calcitonin injection: 0.5 mg/vial.

Usual Adult Doses

Salmon calcitonin injection: For osteoporosis, the usual adult dose is 100 units a day given by subcutaneous injection. For Paget's disease the usual adult dose is 50 to 100 units a day by subcutaneous injection. The frequency of the injections can be decreased according to your response.

Salmon calcitonin—nasal spray: The usual adult dose is one spray (200 IU) a day.

Human calcitonin: For Paget's disease the usual adult starting dose is 0.5 mg a day by subcutaneous injection. The dose that is needed can range from 0.25 mg to 0.5 mg two to three times a week to 0.5 mg twice a day.

Comments

Osteoporosis is a common problem, particularly in women after menopause and in people who take corticosteroids. Osteoporosis is diagnosed by measuring your bone density, often with a type of scan known as a DEXA. The usual program to treat or prevent osteoporosis also includes stopping smoking and alcohol, increasing exercise, and taking calcium supplements and a low dose of vitamin D, often as part of a multivitamin tablet.

A few people can develop antibodies to salmon calcitonin injection after a while and become resistant to it. The nasal spray is much more convenient than the injection. The manufacturer also makes special holders that help people who have arthritis affecting their hands to activate the nose spray. Calcitonin does decrease the risk of fractures in people with osteoporosis, but there is stronger evidence from clinical trials that used estrogen or alendronate. So in people who can take them, estrogen or alendronate is usually preferred above nasal calcitonin.

Don't forget that the aim of treating osteoporosis is to prevent fractures and that many fractures are caused by falls. Simple things can reduce your risk of falling. Some of these may apply to you. Get rid of loose throw rugs and other objects that can trip you, have nonslip surfaces, use a cane if you need one, don't hurry—that telephone can keep ringing—and keep a night-light on so that you can see your way to the bathroom. People with poor vision are more likely to fall, so have your vision checked from time to time. Alcohol and medicines that affect your balance, such as many kinds of sleeping pills, increase your risk of falling. Avoid them if possible.

CALCIUM

Brand Names

CALCIUM CARBONATE: *Alka-Mints, Calci-Chew, Caltrate, Os-Cal, Oyst-Cal 500, Rolaids Calcium Rich, Titralac, Tums, Tums E-X,* and many others.
CALCIUM CITRATE: *Citracal.*
CALCIUM LACTATE: Generic.
CALCIUM PHOSPHATE DIBASIC: Generic.

Drug Family

Calcium tablets are used as a supplement to increase your daily intake of calcium to the recommended amount of 1,500 mg a day.

Families of Arthritis Problems Prescribed For

Calcium supplements are used to prevent and treat bone loss (osteoporosis).

How It Works

Calcium tablets supplement your diet and provide you with enough calcium to maintain your bones.

Avoid

Calcium supplements are usually avoided in people who have kidney stones, a high blood-calcium level, or kidney failure.

Side Effects

Common: Most people have no side effects from calcium tablets, but some find the taste unpleasant, and some get constipated or get gas.

Rare: Calcium supplements rarely cause a high blood-calcium level or kidney stones.

Interactions with Other Drugs

Calcium channel antagonists (Verapamil—*Calan*, Nifedipine—*Procardia,* Diltiazem—*Cardizem*): Very high doses of calcium that increase your blood levels of calcium (something that very seldom happens with calcium supplements) can block the effects of the calcium channel blockers, a group of drugs most often used to treat high blood pressure.

Digoxin (*Lanoxin*): Very high doses of calcium that increase your blood levels of calcium can increase the risk of having an abnormal heart rhythm with digoxin.

Iron tablets: Calcium tablets block the absorption of iron tablets. Do not take calcium and iron tablets within two hours of each other.

Tetracycline antibiotics: Calcium tablets block their absorption. Do not take calcium and tetracyclines within two hours of each other.

Important Information

- Calcium supplements are best taken at meals with a large glass of water. Calcium tablets stop the absorption of many drugs, so wait at least one to two hours after you have taken your other medicines before taking your calcium tablets.
- Calcium supplements need to be taken regularly.

Common Dose Sizes and Usual Adult Doses

The usual dose of calcium to treat or prevent osteoporosis in adults is enough to bring your total daily intake of calcium up to 1 to 1.5 g a day. The different calcium salts provide different amounts of calcium. Virtually all of the calcium preparations that you can buy in the supermarket show how many milligrams of calcium each tablet provides. Some common preparations are shown in the table that follows. If you don't find your preparation in the table, read the label carefully; it will always tell you how much calcium there is in a tablet, and usually how many tablets a day you need to take to get the recommended daily intake.

Comments

Calcium supplements are needed because our modern diet does not provide most of us with enough calcium. There is not much difference between the calcium preparations, and I do not recommend one above another. Calcium is usually given with a low dose of vitamin D (400 IU/day) to improve

CALCIUM TABLETS

Calcium Preparation	*Calcium per tablet (mg)*	*Tablets per day**
Calcium carbonate—*generic*	600 or 500 mg	2
Most of the big drugstores also have their own brands. Go for the cheapest—calcium is calcium.		
Caltrate 600	600	2
Os-Cal 500	500	2
Tums 500	500	2
Calcium carbonate + vitamin D	500 or 600 mg calcium with 125 or 200 units of vitamin D	2
Most of the brand name and generic manufacturers have a product that has 500 mg or 600 mg of calcium combined with 125 or 200 units of vitamin D.		
Caltrate 600 + D		
Oscal + D		
Calcium citrate—*generic*	200	5
Citracal	200	5
Calcium phosphate *Posture-D*	600	2

* The number of tablets a day that will provide you with the recommended daily calcium intake of 1,000 to 1,200 mg of calcium.

its absorption into your body. There are some combination tablets that provide calcium and this amount of vitamin D, and some people find them convenient. Other people prefer to take a multivitamin that contains about 400 IU of vitamin D. Calcium and vitamin D alone help prevent osteoporosis in people who do not get enough calcium and vitamin D in their diets, but on their own they are not enough to treat osteoporosis. For most people with osteoporosis, calcium and vitamin D are the foundation of treatment, and other medicines such as estrogens, selective estrogen receptor modulators, bisphosphonates, or calcitonin are added.

Don't forget that the aim of treating osteoporosis is to prevent fractures and that many fractures are caused by falls. Simple things can reduce your risk of falling. Some of these may apply to you. Get rid of loose throw rugs and other objects that can trip you, have nonslip surfaces, use a cane if you need one, don't hurry—that telephone can keep ringing—and keep a night-light on so that you can see your way to the bathroom. People with poor vision are more likely to fall, so have your vision checked from time to time. Alcohol and medicines that affect your balance, such as many kinds of sleeping pills, increase your risk of falling. Avoid them if possible.

CALTRATE (SEE CALCIUM)

CAPSAICIN

Brand Names

Zostrix, Capsin, Theragen, Trixaicin, and *Capsagel.*

Drug Family

Capsaicin is an analgesic cream or ointment that is rubbed onto painful joints. Capsaicin was developed from the hot stuff that makes chilies hot.

Families of Arthritis Problems Prescribed For

Capsaicin is most often used for painful joints caused by osteoarthritis. It is also used for painful nerve problems that can follow an attack of shingles (herpes zoster) or that happen in some people with nerve damage caused by diabetes.

How It Works

Many "arthritis creams" work as a counterirritant; they make your skin burn, and this blurs the arthritis pain. Capsaicin does not work like this. It affects the nerves that conduct pain signals and lowers the amount of a messenger, called substance P, in these nerves.

Avoid

Do not use capsaicin if you are allergic to it. Do not apply it on areas where you have a rash or broken skin.

Take Precautions

- Make sure the cream does not come into contact with your eyes, mouth, genitals, or an open wound.

Side Effects

Common: The first few times that you apply capsaicin, you may feel a burning sensation. This usually goes away after you have used it for a while. Skin irritation can occur. If capsaicin gets into your eyes, they will burn.

Important Information

- Use capsaicin only on your skin. Do not apply it to broken skin. Use gloves or an applicator to apply it. Wash your hands after using it.
- Capsaicin can provide temporary pain relief, but it does not change the underlying arthritis.

• Capsaicin has to be applied regularly for it to be effective. If you put it on only when you hurt, it will not work.

• The effects come on slowly, and it may take several weeks, or even a month or two, of regular use before you see improvement.

Common Dose Sizes

Many prescription and over-the-counter capsaicin preparations are available in different sizes and strengths.

Cream: 0.025 percent (45 g and 90 g tube), 0.075 percent (30 g and 60 g tube).

Usual Adult Doses

Capsaicin is applied regularly three to four times a day, whether you are hurting or not. If you apply it less often, it is less effective.

Comments

Some people find the burning sensation when they start using capsaicin unpleasant. A lot of people give up when they don't notice any change in pain within a few days. The effects of capsaicin can be delayed for weeks, so do not give up too soon if you are trying capsaicin. In my practice, few people seem to get useful arthritis pain relief from capsaicin, but because it has so few side effects, it may be worth a try. It is most suitable for people who have problems such as osteoarthritis in only a few joints.

CARISOPRODOL

Brand Names

Rela, Soma.

Drug Family

Carisoprodol is a muscle relaxant.

Families of Arthritis Problems Prescribed For

Carisoprodol is often used to treat painful muscle spasms but is also sometimes useful for fibromyalgia.

How It Works

We do not know exactly how carisoprodol works.

Avoid

Do not take carisoprodol if you are allergic to it. Carisoprodol is also avoided in people with a rare problem called acute intermittent porphyria.

Take Precautions

- Caution is needed in people with poor liver or kidney function.

Side Effects

Common: Drowsiness is common.

Less common: Flushing, nausea, vomiting, lightheadedness, feeling stimulated or "hyper," shakiness, and rash.

Rare: Allergy with swelling of the face or tongue, an addiction problem, and bone-marrow problems.

Interactions with Other Drugs

Any other sedative drug: Carisoprodol can make people sleepy, so combining it with any other sedative drug, such as alcohol, can be dangerous.

Important Information

- Don't take more than the prescribed dose.
- Don't drink alcohol while you are taking carisoprodol.

- Carisoprodol can cause drowsiness and affect your concentration for driving and other tasks.

Common Dose Sizes

Tablet: 350 mg.

Usual Adult Doses

The usual dose of carisoprodol in adults who have an acute, short-term problem is one 350 mg tablet taken two to four times a day. For fibromyalgia, a single nighttime dose of 350 mg is often used.

Comments

The sedative effect of carisoprodol is sometimes helpful to improve sleep in fibromyalgia. There is a potential for addiction. Remember, it only treats symptoms. If it doesn't help you, there is no point in taking it.

CELECOXIB

Brand Name

Celebrex.

Drug Family

Celecoxib belongs to the nonsteroidal anti-inflammatory drug (NSAID) family. There are two big groups of NSAIDs, divided by whether they inhibit both cyclo-oxygenase (COX) enzymes, COX-1 and COX-2, or are more selective for COX-2. Celecoxib is selective for COX-2 and has little effect on COX-1.

Families of Arthritis Problems Prescribed For

NSAIDs are used to treat all kinds of pain and inflammation, whether they affect the joints or not. NSAIDs are used to treat many kinds of arthritis problems, such as RA, osteoarthritis, and bursitis. NSAIDs decrease pain and inflammation but do not change the progression of arthritis.

How It Works

Most NSAIDs inhibit the enzymes COX-1 and COX-2, but selective NSAIDs, such as celecoxib, are more selective for COX-2. Inhibiting these cyclo-oxygenase enzymes decreases the formation of chemicals called prostaglandins. Decreasing the prostaglandins made by COX-2 is anti-inflammatory, which is usually why we use NSAIDs. NSAIDs that inhibit COX-1 make platelets in your blood less sticky, which is why aspirin is used to treat heart attacks. COX-1 also protects the stomach from ulcers, so blocking COX-1 may be why the nonselective NSAIDs increase the risk of peptic ulcers. Because celecoxib selectively blocks COX-2, it is kinder on the stomach than nonselective NSAIDs and also does not make platelets less sticky.

Avoid

Do not take celecoxib if you are allergic to it. People who have had a serious allergic reaction (swelling of the face and tongue, and wheezing) to one NSAID can have the same reaction to others. People with asthma or nasal polyps are more likely to be allergic to NSAIDs. You should not take celecoxib if you are allergic to sulfonamides ("sulfa drugs"). NSAIDs are avoided if someone has an active peptic ulcer or is pregnant.

Take Precautions

- NSAIDs can cause fluid retention and can worsen heart failure and high blood pressure.
- Some people have a higher risk for peptic ulcers caused by NSAIDs. Risk factors are being older than 65 years, having

had a previous peptic ulcer, having had a previous bleeding ulcer, and taking a corticosteroid. In people who have a higher risk for peptic ulcers caused by NSAIDs, most rheumatologists would avoid an NSAID, if possible. If this is not possible, then prescribing misoprostol (see MISOPROSTOL—*Cytotec*) or a proton pump inhibitor (see OMEPRAZOLE—*Prilosec*) to protect against peptic ulcers caused by NSAIDs is an option. Another option is to use a COX-2 selective NSAID such as CELECOXIB (*Celebrex*) or ROFECOXIB (*Vioxx*). None of these choices is foolproof, and peptic ulcers can still happen.

• NSAIDs, even COX-2 selective NSAIDs, have to be used carefully in people who have asthma or liver or kidney problems.

• If you are taking NSAIDs regularly, blood tests will be done from time to time to check your blood count (in case you are losing blood slowly from an ulcer that you may not know about), your creatinine (for kidney function), and liver enzymes. People taking diuretics ("water pills") or ACE (angiotensin converting enzyme) inhibitors—a family of drugs that lowers blood pressure—and people with diabetes, heart failure, or existing kidney problems are more likely to have kidney problems caused by NSAIDs. These people may need more frequent blood tests to check their kidney function.

Side Effects

Common: NSAIDs are one of the most common medicines we take. Many people tolerate NSAIDs reasonably well. GI problems, usually indigestion or heartburn, are common reasons why people stop NSAIDs. One of the less common but more severe side effects is a serious peptic ulcer problem. When GI problems are measured by symptoms such as indigestion or by the number of small ulcers seen on endoscopy, celecoxib, one of the selective COX-2 blocking NSAIDs, clearly causes fewer GI problems than nonselective NSAIDs. The risk of serious bleeding from peptic ulcers is probably also lower with selective COX-2 blocking NSAIDs such as celecoxib than it is with nonselective NSAIDs. NSAIDs often cause some fluid retention, with a little ankle swelling.

Less common: Peptic ulcers can be silent, without warning symptoms such as indigestion. Small ulcers occur in many people taking NSAIDs without their even knowing it. In people at higher risk (older than 65 years, a previous peptic ulcer, a previous bleeding ulcer, and combined treatment with a corticosteroid), the annual risk of a serious ulcer problem with nonselective NSAIDs can be as high as three out of every 100 people. It is not yet clear how these numbers apply to selective COX-2 blocking NSAIDs such as celecoxib, but it is likely that the risk will be lower.

Blood pressure can increase in some people, usually by a small amount. Abnormal liver function tests (usually mild), rashes, ringing in the ears, and a feeling of lightheadedness or feeling "spacy" can occur.

Rare: Bleeding from an ulcer, perforation of the bowel, serious liver problems, rash, dizziness, and kidney problems can occur. People who have an allergic reaction to one NSAID and experience wheezing, a lumpy and itchy rash, and swelling of the tongue or face are often allergic to other NSAIDs.

Interactions with Other Drugs

Warfarin (*Coumadin*): Celecoxib, unlike the nonselective NSAIDs, does not make platelets less sticky. Even so, celecoxib is avoided if possible in people taking warfarin or other anticoagulants because there is still a small risk of a peptic ulcer.

NSAIDs: A combination of two NSAIDs is avoided because

it does not improve the control of inflammation but does increase the risk of side effects. But celecoxib has no effects on platelets, so if someone needs aspirin to prevent a heart attack or stroke, a low dose of aspirin is often prescribed with celecoxib.

Lithium: Many NSAIDs, including celecoxib, can increase lithium levels. Lithium levels are usually monitored, and the dose of lithium can be decreased if needed.

Diuretics ("water pills") or ACE (angiotensin converting enzyme) inhibitors—a family of drugs that lowers blood pressure: Many NSAIDs blunt the ability of these drugs to lower blood pressure.

Fluconazole (*Diflucan*): Fluconazole doubles the blood levels of celecoxib. This does not usually cause problems, but lower doses of celecoxib should be used with fluconazole.

Important Information

- The risks of peptic ulcers from NSAIDs are much lower with selective COX-2 inhibitors than they are with nonselective NSAIDs, but remember that peptic ulcers can still occur.
- Taking NSAIDs with food is a good idea and may protect you from indigestion, but it does not prevent peptic ulcers.
- To minimize your GI risks, use the lowest effective dose of an NSAID.
- One of the signs that you may be bleeding from the stomach is if you have pitch-black bowel movements. Bowel movements with altered blood, in addition to being black, are also often runny and very smelly. If this happens, contact your doctor immediately.

Common Dose Sizes

Capsule: 100 mg, 200 mg.

Usual Adult Doses

The usual adult dose of celecoxib is 100 mg twice a day or 200 mg once a day. For some people with RA, 200 mg twice a day is used.

Comments

Most people take NSAIDs for arthritis pain. There is no convincing evidence that one NSAID is more effective than another for arthritis pain. But people respond differently, and you may find that one particular NSAID suits you much better than any of the others. There are many NSAIDs on the market. I don't think there is much point in trying a lot of different NSAIDs to get greater effect. If two or three NSAIDs don't help much, it usually means that some other type of treatment may be better for you.

Some people with osteoarthritis find that NSAIDs and acetaminophen reduce their pain by about the same amount. If this is the case for you, take acetaminophen because it is safer. Rheumatoid arthritis causes a lot more inflammation than osteoarthritis, and NSAIDs usually control the symptoms of RA better than does acetaminophen. People vary a lot. Some people with RA tell me they find that NSAIDs make little difference to their symptom control. For them, the risks outweigh the benefits, and I suggest that they do not take an NSAID. Other people with RA find that NSAIDs help them a lot. RA is virtually never controlled by an NSAID alone, so a DMARD is introduced early in the treatment plan.

There are many unanswered questions about NSAIDs. Do the serious ulcer problems caused by older NSAIDs in relatively few people mean that everyone should be treated with a new COX-2 selective NSAID, although it may cost more? Are there side effects from the new COX-2 selective NSAIDs that we don't know about yet? In people at higher risk for ulcers, are COX-2 selective NSAIDs safer than a nonselective NSAID taken with a stomach protective agent? We don't know the answers to these questions. My approach is not to change people who are stable on their older NSAID to a newer COX-2 selective drug. In people at higher risk for NSAID ulcer problems, I discuss the choices available and use a COX-2 selective drug or an older NSAID with either misoprostol (see MISOPROSTOL—*Cytotec*) or a proton pump inhibitor (see OMEPRAZOLE—*Prilosec*) to protect against ulcers. As more information becomes available, we will have clearer answers to these questions. I suspect that COX-2 selective NSAIDs, because they are equally effective and are likely to be safer, will replace the nonselective NSAIDs as the first choice for most people with arthritis who need NSAIDs.

CELLCEPT (SEE MYCOPHENOLATE MOFETIL)

CHLORAMBUCIL

Brand Names

Leukeran.

Drug Family

Chlorambucil is an anticancer drug that modulates the immune system. It was first used to treat cancer and was then found to be useful for some rheumatic illnesses. Smaller doses are used to treat rheumatic problems than are used to treat cancer. Side effects are less common with the lower doses used in rheumatology than with the doses used for cancer chemotherapy.

Families of Arthritis Problems Prescribed For

Chlorambucil is not used very often anymore. When it is used, it is usually used to suppress the immune system in someone who cannot take cyclophosphamide. Cyclophosphamide (and chlorambucil) are used to treat vasculitis, lupus affecting organs such as the brain or the kidney, and other serious problems. Chlorambucil was tried in RA, but it has been replaced by safer and more effective drugs. It is sometimes used for connective tissue problems affecting the eye, such as Behçet's disease, an uncommon problem that can cause mouth and genital ulcers and eye and joint problems.

How It Works

Chlorambucil interferes with the formation of DNA, particularly in cells such as white blood cells.

Avoid

Do not take chlorambucil if you are allergic to it. Avoid chlorambucil in pregnancy.

Take Precautions

- Your blood count will need to be checked from time to time, often every one to two weeks initially, and then less often once you are on a stable dose of chlorambucil. Liver function tests are also checked, but much less often.
- Chlorambucil suppresses your immune system, so take any infections that you get seriously and have them treated early.
- Caution is needed in people with poor liver or kidney function.

Side Effects

Common: Bone marrow suppression with a drop in the white cell count and/or platelet count is fairly common.

Less common: Rash, GI problems such as nausea, vomiting, and diarrhea, and mouth ulcers are less common.

Rare: Rare side effects are confusion, seizures, changes in the menstrual cycle, infertility, lung scarring, serious liver problems, fever, and increased frequency of cancer.

Interactions with Other Drugs

Other immunosuppressants: All drugs that suppress the immune system increase the risk of side effects such as infection. The more the immune system is suppressed, the higher the risk. High doses of corticosteroids, alone or with other drugs such as chlorambucil, increase the risk of infection.

Live vaccines: Some vaccines are given as a weaker strain of a live virus. These vaccines are usually avoided in people taking drugs that can suppress the immune system.

Important Information

- Avoid becoming pregnant while you are taking chlorambucil.
- Do not take more than the prescribed dose of chlorambucil.
- Regular monitoring of your blood count is important.
- Avoid immunizations (except for influenza and pneumonia immunization) unless discussed with your physician.
- Contact your doctor if you develop any serious or prolonged infection or fever.

Common Dose Sizes

Tablet: 2 mg.

Usual Adult Doses

The usual adult dose of chlorambucil is in the range of 4 mg to 8 mg a day. The dose is adjusted according to your response and your blood count.

Comments

When possible, azathioprine or methotrexate are used in preference to chlorambucil because they are less likely to increase the risk of cancer. Chlorambucil is most often used for people who cannot take cyclophosphamide, because cyclophosphamide has caused vomiting that cannot be easily controlled or bladder side effects.

CHLOROQUINE

(SEE HYDROXYCHLOROQUINE)

CHOLINE MAGNESIUM SALICYLATE

Brand Name

Trilisate.

Drug Family

Choline magnesium salicylate belongs to the NSAID family but belongs to a subfamily called nonacetylated salicylates, which behaves a little differently from other NSAIDs.

Families of Arthritis Problems Prescribed For

Nonacetylated salicylates are used as NSAIDs for rheumatoid arthritis and osteoarthritis. Nonacetylated salicylates are chemically very similar to aspirin but have slight differences in their structure that change the way they work and their side effects.

How It Works

It is not clear how nonacetylated salicylates work. Unlike other NSAIDs, they are only weak inhibitors of the cyclooxygenase (COX) enzymes that make prostaglandins. They may have some of their effect by either blocking or slowing the formation of COX-2.

Avoid

Do not take nonacetylated salicylates if you are allergic to aspirin or other salicylates. People who have had a serious allergic reaction (swelling of the face and tongue, and wheezing) to one NSAID can have the same reaction with other NSAIDs. People with asthma or nasal polyps are more likely to be allergic to NSAIDs. Salicylates are avoided in children, if someone has an active peptic ulcer, is bleeding, or is pregnant.

Take Precautions

• NSAIDs can cause fluid retention and can worsen heart failure and high blood pressure.

• Some people have a higher risk for peptic ulcers caused by NSAIDs. Risk factors are being older than 65 years, having had a previous peptic ulcer, having had a previous bleeding ulcer, and taking a corticosteroid. In people who are at higher risk for peptic ulcers caused by NSAIDs, most rheumatologists would avoid an NSAID, if possible. If this is not possible, then prescribing misoprostol (see MISOPROSTOL—*Cytotec*) or a proton pump inhibitor (see OMEPRAZOLE—*Prilosec*) to protect against peptic ulcers caused by NSAIDs is an option. Another option is to use a COX-2 selective NSAID (see CELECOXIB—*Celebrex* and ROFECOXIB—*Vioxx*). None of these choices is foolproof, and peptic ulcers can still happen.

• Salicylates have to be used carefully in people who have asthma or liver or kidney problems.

• If you are taking NSAIDs regularly, blood tests will be done from time to time to check your blood count (in case you are losing blood slowly from an ulcer that you may not know about), your creatinine (for kidney function), and liver enzymes. People taking diuretics ("water pills") or ACE (angiotensin converting enzyme) inhibitors—a family of drugs that lowers blood pressure—and people with diabetes, heart failure, or existing kidney problems are more likely to have kidney problems caused by NSAIDs. These people may need more frequent blood tests to check their kidney function.

Side Effects

Common: Stomach irritation causing indigestion, heartburn, and pain in the stomach. NSAIDs often cause some fluid retention with a little ankle swelling.

Less common: Peptic ulcers can be silent, without warning symptoms such as indigestion. In people who have a higher risk for peptic ulcer (older than 65 years, a previous peptic ulcer, a previous bleeding ulcer, and taking a corticosteroid), the annual risk of an ulcer problem with aspirin and other nonselective NSAIDs can be as high as three out of every 100 people. The risk is probably lower with nonacetylated salicylates. Salicylates in doses that are too high for you can make your ears ring and affect your hearing.

Rare: Bleeding from an ulcer, perforation of the bowel, and liver and kidney problems can occur. People who are allergic to aspirin and who have wheezing, a lumpy and itchy rash, and swelling of the tongue or face when they take aspirin are often allergic to other NSAIDs. Reye's syndrome is a very rare problem that caused liver failure and coma in children treated with aspirin for a viral illness. It virtually disappeared after the recommendation that aspirin should not be used in children—so other salicylates are also generally avoided in children.

Interactions with Other Drugs

Antacids: Antacids can decrease the effect of salicylates by increasing their excretion in the urine.

Warfarin (*Coumadin*): Salicylates can increase the anticoagulant (anti–blood clotting) effect of warfarin in some people. If you are taking warfarin to prevent blood clots and you start taking a salicylate, you may need to have your blood monitored more frequently than usual, and your dose of warfarin may need to be changed. Nonacetylated salicylates do not affect platelet stickiness.

NSAIDs: A combination of two NSAIDs is avoided because it does not improve control of inflammation but does increase the risk of side effects. But if someone on an NSAID needs aspirin to prevent a heart attack or stroke, a low dose of aspirin is often prescribed with the other NSAID.

Methotrexate: Aspirin, other salicylates, and other NSAIDs can increase the concentrations of methotrexate, usually by a small amount. In rheumatology practice, with the low doses of methotrexate used, this interaction is seldom important, and methotrexate is often prescribed with an NSAID for RA.

Lithium: Many NSAIDs can increase lithium levels. Lithium levels are usually monitored and the dose of lithium can be decreased if needed.

Diuretics ("water pills") or ACE (angiotensin converting enzyme) inhibitors—a family of drugs that lowers blood pressure): Many NSAIDs blunt the ability of these drugs to lower blood pressure.

Important Information

- Taking NSAIDs with food is a good idea and may protect you from indigestion, but it does not prevent peptic ulcers.
- Nonacetylated salicylates have little effect on platelet stickiness.
- One of the signs that you may be bleeding from the stomach is if you have pitch-black bowel movements. Bowel movements with altered blood, in addition to being black, are also often runny and very smelly. If this happens, contact your doctor immediately.

Common Dose Sizes

Tablets: 500 mg, 750 mg, and 1,000 mg.

Usual Adult Doses

The usual adult dose of choline magnesium salicylate is 2 to 4 g a day, split into three doses.

Comments

Nonacetylated salicylate are salicylates like aspirin, but their different chemical structure makes them behave more like COX-2 selective NSAIDs so that they have little effect on platelet stickiness and are kinder on the stomach. Some patients find that they are not as effective as other NSAIDs for controlling their arthritis symptoms. Nonacetylated salicylates are a useful option for people who have stomach problems with NSAIDs or are at high risk for NSAIDs causing stomach ulcers.

CHONDROITIN SULFATE

(SEE GLUCOSAMINE)

CIMETIDINE

Brand Name

Tagamet.

Drug Family.

Cimetidine belongs to a family of drugs called H_2-receptor antagonists, or H_2-blockers, that decrease acid production by the stomach.

Families of Arthritis Problems Prescribed For

Cimetidine is not used to treat arthritis but is often used to treat the GI side effects that can result from some arthritis medicines, particularly NSAIDs. H_2-receptor antagonists are used to treat and prevent peptic ulcers and esophageal reflux symptoms.

How It Works

H_2-receptor antagonists block histamine receptors in the stomach and decrease acid production.

Avoid

Do not take cimetidine if you are allergic to it.

Take Precautions

- Cimetidine interacts with many other medicines. Newer H_2-receptor antagonists have fewer drug interactions.
- H_2-receptor antagonists, except in high doses, are not effective protection against peptic ulcers caused by NSAIDs.

Side Effects

H_2-receptor antagonists are very well tolerated and few people have to stop them because of side effects.

Common: Minor, transient problems such as dizziness, headache, and diarrhea can occur.

Rare: Increased breast tissue with swelling of the breasts in men (called gynecomastia), rash, liver, muscle, and blood problems are uncommon.

Interactions with Other Drugs

Cimetidine slows the breakdown of many drugs. So if you are taking one of these drugs and start taking cimetidine, you can have higher blood levels of the drug than you would normally have. For some drugs in which a small change in blood levels can be important, such as theophylline and warfarin, it is safer to take one of the other H_2-receptor antagonists. These have fewer drug interactions.

Some of the drugs whose levels are increased when they

are given with cimetidine are Warfarin (*Coumadin*), Theophylline (*Theo-Dur* and many others), Phenytoin (*Dilantin*), Quinidine (*Quinaglute* and others), Propranolol (*Inderal* and others), Tricyclic antidepressants (see AMITRIPTYLINE), and Cyclosporine (*Neoral, Sandimmune*).

Important Information

- H_2-receptor antagonists may decrease the GI symptoms caused by NSAIDs, but peptic ulcers can still occur.

Common Dose Sizes

Tablet: 200 mg, 300 mg, 400 mg, 800 mg.

Usual Adult Doses

To treat an active peptic ulcer, the usual adult dose of cimetidine is 400 mg twice a day. To stop ulcers from coming back, 400 mg at night is often used.

Comments

Cimetidine is on many formularies because it is sometimes cheaper than other H_2-receptor antagonists. If there is no cost difference, I use one of the newer H_2-receptor antagonists (see the table that follows) because they have fewer drug interactions.

PROFILES OF COMMON H_2-RECEPTOR ANTAGONIST DRUGS

Generic Name	*Brand Name*	*Adult Dose*
Cimetidine	*Tagamet*	800 mg a day to treat an ulcer, 400 mg a day to prevent an ulcer
Famotidine	*Pepcid*	40 mg a day to treat an ulcer, 20 mg a day to prevent an ulcer
Nizatidine	*Axid*	300 mg a day to treat an ulcer, 150 mg a day to prevent an ulcer
Ranitidine	*Zantac*	300 mg a day to treat an ulcer, 150 mg a day to prevent an ulcer

CISAPRIDE

Brand Name
Propulsid.

Drug Family
Cisapride stimulates movement of the muscles in the stomach and small intestine.

Families of Arthritis Problems Prescribed For
Cisapride is not used to treat any arthritis problem directly, but it is used in people who have poor motility of their esophagus (the food pipe that joins your mouth to your stomach), stomach, or small intestine. This can happen in scleroderma. Cisapride was sometimes used to treat people with GERD (gastroesophageal reflux disease), which causes reflux of acid and food up the esophagus (the food pipe that joins your mouth to your stomach), but in early 2000, because of serious side effects, it was withdrawn from the general market. The use of cisapride is now restricted to a few patients who do not respond to other drugs.

How It Works
Cisapride causes an increase in the concentrations of a chemical messenger, acetylcholine, in the bowel wall, and this stimulates the bowel muscle.

Avoid
Do not take cisapride if you are allergic to it or if you have serious heart, liver, or lung problems. People who have a blockage in the bowel should not take cisapride. There are many drugs that slow down the metabolism of cisapride. Cis-

apride should not be taken with these drugs (see Interactions with Other Drugs).

Take Precautions

• Care is needed in people who have certain heart-rhythm problems or problems with a low level of potassium or magnesium in their blood.

• Many drugs can interact with cisapride in a potentially dangerous way. If you take cisapride, get a copy of the package insert that comes with the drug so that you can check (and also ask your doctor to check) for drug interactions between your medicines.

Side Effects

Common: Rash, stomach cramps, diarrhea, and gas are common but not serious.

Less common: Nervousness, vomiting, and drowsiness are less common.

Rare: Cisapride has rarely caused a serious type of heart-rhythm problem called *torsades des pointes*. This has usually happened when cisapride has been taken in overdose, or when it was taken with another drug that slowed its breakdown (see Interactions with Other Drugs).

Interactions with Other Drugs

Many drugs block the enzyme that breaks down cisapride. This can lead to high levels of cisapride that have rarely been associated with fatal heart-rhythm problems. Many drugs can increase cisapride levels. The list below is not complete.

Drugs that may increase cisapride levels

Antifungal drugs such as ketoconazole (*Nizoral*), fluconazole (*Diflucan*), itraconazole (*Sporanox*), and miconazole

(*Monistat*). Some antibiotics such as erythromycin (*E.E.S, Erythrocin,* many others), clarithromycin (*Biaxin*), and troleandeomycin (*TAO*).

Some drugs used to treat HIV infection such as indinavir (*Crixivan*), ritonavir (*Norvir*), and others.

Some antidepressants: Nefazodone (*Serzone*).

Some GI drugs: Cimetidine (*Tagamet*).

Grapefruit juice increases cisapride levels. I advise people to avoid it.

Drugs that can act together with cisapride to prolong the QT interval

Cisapride can prolong the QT interval—a measurement on the electrocardiograph (ECG). A very long QT interval is a risk for a serious abnormal heart rhythm called *torsades des pointes*. Many other drugs can also prolong the QT interval, and these are avoided in people taking cisapride. Some of these are:

Many drugs used to treat heart rhythm problems: Quinidine (*Quinaglute, Dura-Tabs,* many others), procainamide (*Procan, Pronestyl*), and sotalol (*Betapace*).

Many tricyclic and other antidepressants (see AMITRIPTYLINE).

Many drugs used to treat schizophrenia.

Other drug interactions with cisapride

Warfarin (*Coumadin*): Cisapride can increase the anticoagulant (anti-blood clotting) effect of warfarin in some people. If you are taking warfarin to prevent blood clots and start taking cisapride, you may need to have your blood monitored more frequently than usual, and your dose of warfarin may need to be changed.

Important Information

- Because of serious side effects, cisapride is now prescribed only for selected patients.
- Do not take more cisapride than is prescribed.
- Do not share cisapride with anyone else.
- Tell every physician that prescribes a new medicine for you that you are taking cisapride.
- Check that any medication prescribed for you does not interact with cisapride. You need to keep a copy of the cisapride package insert with you.
- Do not drink grapefruit juice while you are taking cisapride.

Common Dose Sizes

Tablet: 10 mg.

Usual Adult Doses

The usual adult dose of cisapride is one 10 mg tablet taken fifteen minutes before meals and before bedtime.

Comments

The potential for rare, but very serious, heart-rhythm problems if cisapride is taken together with other commonly used drugs makes me very cautious about prescribing it. In some people with scleroderma affecting the bowel, cisapride can help constipation or reflux a lot. I prefer not to use cisapride for GERD because proton pump inhibitors (see OMEPRAZOLE) usually work well.

CLINORIL (SEE SULINDAC)

CODEINE

Brand Names

Codeine is most often prescribed by its generic name or in a combination analgesic.

Sometimes Called

Codeine sulfate, codeine phosphate.

Drug Family

Codeine is a narcotic analgesic (painkiller).

Families of Arthritis Problems Prescribed For

Codeine is used for moderate to severe pain, whatever the cause. Narcotic analgesics are usually prescribed only for pain that is not controlled by acetaminophen alone or an NSAID alone. Narcotics do not affect inflammation. Usually, codeine is prescribed as a combination preparation with acetaminophen (see ACETAMINOPHEN + NARCOTICS). Codeine also suppresses coughing.

How It Works

Narcotics decrease pain by acting through specific receptors in the brain.

Avoid

Do not take codeine if you are allergic to it. Real allergic reactions are rare, but a lot of people get side effects, such as nausea or feeling "spacy," from codeine. Avoid codeine if you have had an addiction problem.

Take Precautions

- Do not drink alcohol while you are taking narcotics.

• There is a risk of becoming addicted to narcotics. Take the tablets only for pain. If possible, limit the dose and how long you take them.

• Caution is needed in people with poor liver or kidney function.

Side Effects

Side effects with codeine are common but usually mild. People vary in their sensitivity to different narcotics. People who cannot take medicines that contain codeine, for example, may be able to take other preparations containing hydrocodone, and vice versa.

Common: Nausea, vomiting, constipation, poor appetite, dizziness, lightheadedness, or feeling "spacy," and sleepiness are common but not serious.

Less common: An allergic reaction with rash, hives, or asthma is uncommon. Confusion, feeling nervous or agitated, sleeping badly, feeling "high," an addiction problem (trying to get higher doses of narcotic, not to control pain but to feel good), are uncommon but do occur.

Interactions with Other Drugs

Any other sedative drug: Narcotics make people sleepy, and an overdose can make people unconscious. Combining a narcotic with another sedative drug, such as alcohol, can be dangerous.

Cigarette smoking: Decreases the effect of codeine.

Important Information

• Don't take more than the prescribed dose.

• Don't drink alcohol while you are taking narcotic painkillers.

• Narcotics can cause drowsiness and affect your concentration when driving and performing other tasks.

• Codeine is a narcotic and can be addictive (see Comments).

• Narcotics are dangerous in overdose. Keep them away from children.

Common Dose Sizes

Tablet: 15 mg, 30 mg, and 60 mg.

Usual Adult Doses

The usual adult dose of codeine is 15 to 30 mg taken every four to six hours, if needed, to control pain.

Comments

There is some controversy about how narcotic analgesics should be used to control chronic "benign" pain, meaning chronic pain not caused by cancer. This is particularly true for the strong narcotics such as morphine but to a lesser extent is also true for the combination tablets that contain weaker narcotics such as codeine. Some physicians think that the risk of addiction and abuse is too high and limit narcotic prescriptions to short periods, such as a few days, in all patients. Others are less rigid and believe that these analgesics can make life bearable for some people with chronic arthritis pain that cannot be controlled by other strategies. For example, I find them helpful to control pain at night in some people with severe osteoarthritis pain who cannot take NSAIDs because of their side effects. Most rheumatologists do not prescribe narcotics for fibromyalgia because they are not particularly helpful and because they can worsen the sleep disturbance.

Addiction to an analgesic such as codeine is seldom a problem if it is used to control pain. A clue to addictive behavior is if you are trying to get bigger doses of the drug and are not using the bigger doses to control pain. The risk of addiction is higher in people who themselves, or whose family members, have had an addiction problem (alcohol or drugs). I have a few rules for my patients about narcotic prescriptions.

1. Use the tablets only for pain, not to feel good.
2. If you don't have pain, don't take them.
3. Get all your narcotic prescriptions from one doctor and from one pharmacy.
4. Escalating the dose of narcotic can be an early sign of a problem.
5. Never sell, swap, or hoard tablets.
6. If you are in the position of wanting to fool doctors or do illegal things, such as forging signatures to get narcotic prescriptions, then things are way out of control and you need to speak with your physician about getting help.

COLCHICINE

Brand Names
Colchicine is usually prescribed by the generic name.

Drug Family
Colchicine is an antigout drug. Colchicine prevents and treats inflammation, but it does not lower uric acid levels—the underlying problem in gout.

Families of Arthritis Problems Prescribed For
Colchicine is used to suppress and treat acute attacks of gout. It is also used to treat a rare condition called Familial Mediterranean Fever.

How It Works

We are not sure exactly how colchicine works, but it may change the way white blood cells move to an inflamed area.

Avoid

Do not take colchicine if you are allergic to it. Colchicine is avoided in pregnancy and in people with very poor liver or kidney function.

Take Precautions

- Caution is needed in people with poor liver or kidney function.

Side Effects

Common: Colchicine often causes nausea, vomiting, diarrhea, and stomach cramps, particularly when people are taking high doses such as those that are used to treat an acute attack of gout.

Less common: Decreased appetite and mild hair loss are less common.

Rare: Nerve damage, muscle damage, rash, bone marrow problems, liver problems, and decreased sperm count are uncommon.

Interactions with Other Drugs

Cyclosporine (*Sandimmune, Neoral*): There is an increased risk of kidney and muscle problems when colchicine is given with cyclosporine.

Cimetidine (*Tagamet*), erythromycin (*EES, Erythrocin,* and others), tolbutamide (*Orinase*): All of these can increase colchicine blood levels.

Important Information

- Stop colchicine if you suffer nausea or vomiting.

Common Dose Sizes

Tablets: 0.5 mg, 0.6 mg.

Usual Adult Doses

Acute gout attack: The usual adult dose of colchicine for an acute attack of gout is one 0.5 mg or 0.6 mg tablet taken every couple of hours until the pain is relieved or until a maximum of 6 mg has been taken. Colchicine makes most people sick to their stomach before this, usually after they have taken a couple of milligrams.

To suppress gout: The usual adult dose of colchicine to suppress future attacks of gout is 0.5 mg or 0.6 mg once or twice a day.

Comments

I generally prefer NSAIDs to colchicine for treating an acute attack of gout. The sooner in the attack colchicine is taken, the more likely it is to work. Once an acute attack has lasted for a day or two, colchicine is not particularly helpful. Colchicine is helpful for suppressing future attacks of gout in people who have frequent attacks. When someone starts treatment with a drug such as allopurinol to lower their uric acid level, there is a greater chance of an acute attack during the first few months of this treatment. Colchicine (or an NSAID) is used to prevent attacks of gout in people who have just started treatment with allopurinol.

COLLAGEN

Sometimes Called

Chicken collagen.

Families of Arthritis Problems Prescribed For

Collagen has been studied as a treatment for rheumatoid arthritis. It is not approved by the FDA. Most studies in humans have found that collagen treatment does not work for RA.

How It Works

The theory and the science behind collagen treatment are interesting. The idea is that collagen taken by mouth exposes the immune system in your gut to collagen and makes your immune system more tolerant of your own collagen, such as the collagen in the cartilage of your joints. This theory is similar to the theory behind "allergy shots" that desensitize your body's allergic responses. Collagen treatment, so far, is not an effective treatment for RA.

Comments

There are still studies being done testing collagen treatment for RA. Perhaps they will help us find a dose or way of giving collagen that works. The evidence so far does not support a role for collagen treatment in RA.

CORTICOSTEROIDS

Brand Names

There are many different corticosteroid preparations, and they are used for different jobs. It is easiest to divide them into tablets, intravenous and intramuscular injections, and intra-articular injections.

Tablets: PREDNISONE: *Deltasone, Orasone;* METHYLPREDNISOLONE: *Medrol;* DEXAMETHASONE: *Dexone*

Injections: METHYLPREDNISOLONE: *SoluMedrol;* HYDROCORTISONE: *Solu-Cortef;* DEXAMETHASONE: *Decadron*

Intra-articular injections: METHYLPREDNISOLONE ACE-

TATE: *DepoMedrol;* TRIAMCINOLONE: *Aristocort, Aristospan, Kenalog*

Sometimes Called

Corticosteroids are also called glucocorticoids, or sometimes just "steroids." Corticosteroids are related to cortisone, one of the hormones made by our adrenal glands, and are very different from the "steroids" that you read about athletes taking.

Drug Family

These drugs all belong to the corticosteroid family.

Families of Arthritis Problems Prescribed For

Corticosteroids are very effective for controlling inflammation. They are used in many different ways, with different goals.

- **Very high dose intravenous "pulse" corticosteroids**

Very high doses of "pulse" corticosteroids are usually used in situations where the need for treatment is urgent, such as serious vasculitis or systemic lupus erythematosus or to treat severe rheumatoid arthritis that does not respond to other treatments.

- **Oral "dose packs" or long-acting, intramuscular depot corticosteroids**

For people who have a flare of an inflammatory arthritis or who have inflammation in other organs caused by a problem such as lupus, a corticosteroid tablet "dose pack," or else an intramuscular injection of a long-acting depot corticosteroid, will often suppress the symptoms quickly.

- **Oral high-dose corticosteroids**

High doses of corticosteroids, such as 40 mg to 60 mg of prednisone a day, can be used to get control of serious problems such as vasculitis, lupus affecting organs such as the kidneys or brain, and dermatomyositis or polymyositis. Another drug such as cyclophosphamide, methotrexate, or azathioprine is often used in combination with the steroid.

- **Oral low-dose corticosteroids**

People with vasculitis or lupus who started taking high doses of prednisone will, over time, cut back on their dose and may end up taking a low daily dose to help keep their problem controlled.

Many people with rheumatoid arthritis take low doses of corticosteroids, usually less than 7.5 mg of prednisone a day, often for many years. In RA, steroids are usually used in combination with other medicines, such as DMARDs, to help suppress inflammation.

- **Corticosteroids injected into a joint or bursa**

In rheumatoid arthritis, other inflammatory types of arthritis, and osteoarthritis, a long-acting depot corticosteroid is sometimes helpful when it is injected into a swollen joint. This is called an intra-articular injection, *intra* meaning "in" and *articular* meaning "joint." Tendinitis and bursitis can also sometimes be helped by an injection into the bursa or around a tendon.

How It Works

Corticosteroids have strong anti-inflammatory effects and suppress the immune response.

Avoid

Although corticosteroids are often used to treat allergic reactions, there are a few people who are allergic to certain preparations of corticosteroids.

Take Precautions

• Corticosteroids can make the control of diabetes more difficult. The higher the dose of steroid, the worse the diabetes control can be.

• Corticosteroids suppress the immune system in a dose-related way. The higher the dose, the more the immune system is suppressed. Avoid infections. Make sure you get your flu shot and treat any infections early.

• Caution is needed in people with atherosclerosis (hardening of the arteries), hypertension (high blood pressure), any infection, an active peptic ulcer, and liver problems.

• If you take NSAIDs and steroids, your risk of getting a peptic ulcer caused by the NSAIDs is higher. Some preventive treatment may be needed.

• Corticosteroids cause osteoporosis, again, in a dose-related way. If you are taking corticosteroids for a long time, it is wise to make sure that you get enough calcium and vitamin D (see CALCIUM) to protect your bones against osteoporosis. Even so, osteoporosis remains a risk, particularly in people taking more than 5 mg of prednisone a day for a long time. A DEXA scan to measure your bone density may help your doctor decide if you need an additional drug to treat osteoporosis.

• If you have been on steroids for more than a month or two, your own body may not be able to produce enough cortisone, particularly when you are very ill or having surgery. The speed at which your body recovers its ability to make cortisone varies a lot, but it can take months, or even up to a year after you have stopped corticosteroid treatment. Do not stop long-term steroid treatment suddenly. If you are having surgery or are being admitted to the hospital, make sure your doctors know that you have been on steroids.

Side Effects

The side effects of steroids given into the joint and steroids taken as tablets are different.

The side effects of intra-articular steroid injections.

When a long-acting steroid is injected into a swollen joint, your body gets only a small total dose of steroid. Steroid injections into joints have very few side effects. Most of the side effects from intra-articular steroids are from the injection itself and not from the steroid. There is a very small risk, approximately one in 1,000, of an infection getting into a joint when it is injected. Steroid shots can sometimes make the pain and swelling in the joint worse for a day or two, but then things usually improve. If you get a red, hot, swollen joint with fever and chills a few days after an injection into that joint, you should contact your doctor immediately because you may have an infection in the joint. There is also a worry that steroid shots into a joint may damage cartilage and make ligaments weak. So as a general rule, the number of shots you have into any one joint is kept to a minimum.

The side effects of oral corticosteroids.

The side effects of steroids are directly related to the dose you take. It is hard to give you an idea how often side effects happen because the higher the dose of steroid and the longer you take it, the more side effects there will be. Everyone who takes 60 mg of prednisone a day for more than a few weeks will have side effects, but many people who take 5 mg a day, often for years, have few or no side effects.

Common: Steroids, even in low doses, can increase your appetite and you may gain weight. High doses of corticosteroids can make your face round (moon face) and give you a lot of fat around your shoulders and chest. Our skin becomes thin as we age, and steroids make it even thinner. People on steroids bruise and tear their skin more easily. Another common side effect is that steroids can make people feel different. Some people feel stimulated, awake and energetic, but others can be too energetic and talkative, with sleeplessness and mood swings. Other people can become depressed or feel "spacy." This can be a big problem for some people, particularly if they need to take high doses of steroids.

Steroids increase the risk of infections. These can be regular infections such as pneumonia, but can also be less common infections such as tuberculosis. Low doses of steroid, say, less than 10 mg of prednisone a day, probably do not increase the risk of infection much.

Steroids cause osteoporosis (thinning of the bones) and so increase the risk of breaking a bone. Again, this is more of a problem if high doses of steroids are taken for a long time, but even low doses of steroids can cause osteoporosis.

Corticosteroids increase the white cell count in your blood. If the doctors looking after you don't think of this, they may become worried about the high white blood cell count and start a workup for infection—which is another cause of a high white cell count.

Less common: There is an uncommon problem called avascular necrosis, sometimes abbreviated to AVN, that happens more often in people who are taking steroids. This is an uncommon problem, but people with lupus who are taking high doses of steroids seem to have a higher risk of getting it. AVN can happen in people taking steroids for other reasons, and it can even happen in people who have never taken steroids. AVN often starts as a very painful hip, and it is caused by part of the bone not getting enough blood. A small part of the bone can die and deform the hip shape, leading to arthritis in the hip. AVN in the early stages is sometimes treated by surgery to decrease the pressure in the hip. Late AVN may require joint replacement.

Other problems with steroids are high blood pressure, high blood sugar so that some people get sugar diabetes, low potassium, cataracts, weak thigh muscles, and suppressing of the body's own steroid production.

Interactions with Other Drugs

There are a few drugs that increase the speed at which your liver breaks down steroids. So if you are taking rifampin (*Rifadin, Rimactane*), phenytoin (*Dilantin*), or phenobarbitone (*Barbita*), you may need higher doses of steroids.

Diuretics ("water pills"): Both diuretics and corticosteroids can cause you to lose potassium; the combination makes it more likely that your blood potassium level may become low.

NSAIDs: The risk of peptic ulcer is increased when steroids and NSAIDs are combined. However, many people with RA and other problems take NSAIDs and corticosteroids. In people who have a higher risk for peptic ulcers caused by NSAIDs, most rheumatologists would consider prescribing misoprostol (see MISOPROSTOL—*Cytotec*) or a proton pump inhibitor (see OMEPRAZOLE—*Prilosec*) to protect against peptic ulcers caused by NSAIDs. Another option is to use a COX-2 selective NSAID such as CELECOXIB (*Celebrex*) or ROFECOXIB (*Vioxx*). None of these choices is foolproof, and peptic ulcers can still develop.

Important Information

• Take corticosteroids as instructed. Do not experiment with the dose.

• Tell all your physicians that you are on steroids. If you are taking high doses for a long time, consider getting a medical bracelet that has the information that you are taking corticosteroids on it.

• If you have been taking corticosteroids for a while, do not stop taking them suddenly. Not only will your arthritis problem flare, but your body may not be able to make enough of its own cortisone to cope.

• Watch your diet to prevent weight gain. Keep your calorie, sugar, and fat intake down, but make sure you get enough calcium in your diet.

Common Dose Sizes

Tablets: Prednisone—1 mg, 5 mg, 10 mg, 20 mg; Methylprednisolone—2 mg, 4 mg, 8 mg, 16 mg, 24 mg; Dexamethasone—0.25 mg, 0.5 mg, 0.75 mg, 1 mg, 2 mg, 4 mg.

Usual Adult Doses

The dose of corticosteroids people take varies a lot depending on the goals of treatment. Prednisone is the tablet preparation used most often. Prednisone, and another preparation called prednisolone, are very similar in strength and effects. A different type of corticosteroid, dexamethasone, has the same anti-inflammatory effects as prednisone, but dexamethasone is more "concentrated," and smaller doses are used. The smaller doses of dexamethasone have the same effects and side effects as bigger doses of prednisone, and there is no advantage to using dexamethasone. Low doses of prednisone are 10 mg a day or less, and high doses are 40 mg a day or more. Because the side effects of corticosteroids increase with the dose and duration of treatment, we try to use the lowest dose that will control the problem.

The dose of intra-articular depot steroid injected into a joint is decided by your doctor and depends on the size of the joint.

Comments

No group of drugs causes as many strong feelings as do corticosteroids. Everyone has heard about steroids and their "terrible side effects." If you have read through all the side effects, you will be wondering why anyone takes steroids. The reason is that steroids are one of the most effective drugs that we have for controlling inflammation. In some people, steroids save lives or save vital organ function. There is a lot of controversy about the safety of low doses (10 mg a day or less of prednisone) in treating rheumatoid arthritis. In the U.K. and Canada, prednisone is seldom used to treat RA, but in the U.S. about half the people with RA in most rheumatology practices are taking low doses of prednisone with their other medicines. I use steroids in RA, almost always with a DMARD, and find them very helpful to get control of the inflammation. Interestingly, recent evidence shows that corticosteroids may slow the destructive effects of RA on the joint. Over the long term I try to select the people who seem to benefit from the corticosteroid and who get worse as we slowly cut the dose. In RA we try to keep the dose as low as possible, almost always less than 7.5 mg a day of prednisone, and use DMARDs to get control of the RA. Other than a 5 pound weight gain and an increased risk of cataracts, I don't think that prednisone in a dose of 5 mg a day or less causes significant side effects in most people—provided they have an adequate intake of calcium and vitamin D.

Using corticosteroids safely and effectively is part of the art of rheumatology. Here you will benefit from having a rheumatologist. I think that anyone who is taking corticosteroids regularly for an arthritis problem should be seeing a rheumatologist. Non-rheumatologists sometimes use very high doses of prednisone for too long without introducing another therapy to control the arthritis problem.

Corticosteroids are usually taken as a single dose once a

day, most often in the morning. Taking them at night is not usually a good idea because they keep some people awake. But a few people like to take some of their steroid dose at night because they feel the nighttime dose helps their pain at night. When people need a dose of prednisone above 20 mg a day, I usually split the dose and have them take it twice a day because a split dose seems less likely to make people stimulated or "hyper."

Weight gain can be a big problem, even with low doses of steroids. Corticosteroids can stimulate your appetite, so you have to keep a very close eye on what you are eating.

High doses of steroids or steroids that are needed for only a few weeks can often be cut back fairly quickly, in 10 mg or 5 mg steps, but when doctors are trying to cut back the dose in people who have been taking steroids for a long time, they sometimes reduce the dose too quickly. If someone has been on a dose of 10 mg or less of prednisone for a long time and we are planning to cut back, I usually cut back in 1 mg steps. In other words, from 5 mg to 4 mg. Then, if things are going well, we cut back again by another 1 mg in a few weeks, and so on.

CUPRIMINE (SEE PENICILLAMINE)

CYCLOBENZAPRINE

Brand Names

Cycoflex, Flexeril

Drug Family

Cyclobenzaprine belongs to the muscle-relaxer family.

Families of Arthritis Problems Prescribed For

Cyclobenzaprine is often used to treat painful muscle spasms but is sometimes useful for fibromyalgia.

How It Works

We do not know exactly how cyclobenzaprine works. It is related to the tricyclic antidepressants (see AMITRIPTYLINE).

Avoid

Do not take cyclobenzaprine if you are allergic to it. Do not use cyclobenzaprine within fourteen to twenty-one days of taking a monoamine oxidase inhibitor type of antidepressant. Cyclobenzaprine is avoided soon after a heart attack.

Take Precautions

- Cyclobenzaprine may cause you to be sleepy and may affect your ability to drive or to operate machinery.
- Men who have prostate trouble may find that it becomes more difficult to pass urine.
- Dry eyes and dry mouth, which are problems in Sjogren's syndrome, can get worse.
- Cyclobenzaprine can bring on glaucoma (high blood pressure in the eyeball), particularly in people who are already predisposed to it.

Side Effects

Common: Sleepiness is common, and cyclobenzaprine is often used to improve sleep. Cyclobenzaprine can cause your mouth and eyes to feel dry, blur the vision slightly, cause constipation, and particularly in men with prostate problems, cause some difficulty passing urine. These side effects are called "anticholinergic" side effects. You may find that your body gets used to some of these side effects and you notice them less as you take cyclobenzaprine for a longer time.

Less common: Many people have some drowsiness when

they take cyclobenzaprine, but some people find the opposite. Dizziness when standing up suddenly, tremor (shakiness), nausea, confusion, and stomach upset can occur

Rare: Rarer side effects are heart-rhythm problems, a rash, and liver problems.

Interactions with Other Drugs

Alcohol and other sedatives: These increase the sedative effects of cyclobenzaprine.

Tricyclic antidepressants (see AMITRIPTYLINE): The risk of anticholinergic side effects is increased with this combination.

Monoamine oxidase inhibitor antidepressants—Isocarboxazid (*Marplan*), Phenelzine (*Nardil*), Tranylcypromine (*Parnate*): There is an increased risk of serious heart and blood pressure side effects and even death if these drugs are taken at the same time or within a few weeks of taking cyclobenzaprine.

Guanethidine (*Ismelin*), Guanadrel (*Hylorel*), and Clonidine (*Catapres*): Cyclobenzaprine can block the blood-pressure-lowering effects of these antihypertensive drugs.

Important Information

- Don't take more than the prescribed dose of cyclobenzaprine.
- Don't drink alcohol while you are taking cyclobenzaprine.
- Cyclobenzaprine may cause drowsiness and affect your concentration when driving and performing other tasks.

Common Dose Sizes

Tablet: 10 mg.

Usual Adult Doses

The usual adult dose of cyclobenzaprine is one or two 10 mg tablets taken at night, or else one 10 mg tablet taken twice a day.

Comments

The sedative effect of cyclobenzaprine is sometimes helpful to improve sleep in fibromyalgia. It only treats symptoms. If it doesn't help you, there is no point in taking it.

CYCLOPHOSPHAMIDE

Brand Names

Cytoxan, Neosar.

Drug Family

Cyclophosphamide is an anticancer drug that modulates the immune system. Cyclophosphamide was first used to treat cancer and was then found to be useful for some rheumatic illnesses. Smaller doses of cyclophosphamide are used to treat rheumatic problems than are used to treat cancer, and side effects are less common than in cancer chemotherapy.

Families of Arthritis Problems Prescribed For

Cyclophosphamide, almost always with a corticosteroid such as prednisone, is most often used to get a problem such as vasculitis, or lupus affecting the kidneys or another important organ, into remission. Cyclophosphamide helps prevent damage to the kidneys or other organs that problems such as lupus and vasculitis can cause. Cyclophosphamide was tried in RA, but it has been replaced by safer and more effective drugs. It is sometimes used for connective-tissue problems affecting the eye, such as Behçet's disease, an uncommon problem that can cause mouth and genital ulcers and eye and joint problems.

How It Works

Cyclophosphamide interferes with the formation of DNA, particularly in cells such as white blood cells.

Avoid

Do not take cyclophosphamide if you are allergic to it. Cyclophosphamide is avoided in pregnancy.

Take Precautions

- Your blood count will need to be checked from time to time, often every one to two weeks initially, and then less often once you are on a stable dose of cyclophosphamide. Liver function tests are also checked, but much less often.
- Cyclophosphamide suppresses your immune system, so take seriously any infections that you get and have them treated early.
- Caution is needed in people with poor liver or kidney function.
- Take cyclophosphamide in the morning. Drink plenty of liquids, and empty your bladder frequently during the day. Doing these two things will dilute the concentrations of the breakdown product of cyclophosphamide in your urine that causes bladder damage.
- If you have had to take cyclophosphamide tablets for a long time, you will need to have your urine checked regularly, even after you have stopped the cyclophosphamide. This is done as a preventive check against bladder cancer.

Side Effects

The side effects of cyclophosphamide are a little different depending on whether it is given as a daily tablet or as a monthly intravenous injection. The big advantage of the monthly IV injection is that it almost never causes serious bladder problems. It may also have slightly less effect on fertility and cause a slightly lower risk of infection.

Common: Stomach upset with nausea and vomiting is common but can usually be controlled with medicines.

Less common: Some side effects of cyclophosphamide increase with the dose you take, how much it suppresses your white blood cell count, and how long you take it.

Cyclophosphamide suppresses the bone marrow that makes blood cells so that the white blood cell count and platelet count can drop too low. After an IV injection, the white blood cell counts are lowest about two weeks after the injection, and by three to four weeks after the injection, the counts have usually gone back to normal. Cyclophosphamide increases the risk of infections. These can be regular infections, such as pneumonia, but can also be less common infections, such as tuberculosis. This risk is higher in people who need to take high doses of corticosteroids with cyclophosphamide.

Cyclophosphamide is broken down to a chemical that is very irritating to the bladder. This chemical can cause bladder irritation with burning, needing to pass urine more frequently, and even severe bleeding from the bladder. To try to dilute the toxic chemical in your urine, you may be asked to keep your urine dilute by drinking a lot of fluids immediately before and for several hours after you take your dose. Over many years cyclophosphamide increases the risk of bladder cancer, skin cancer, and blood cancers.

Cyclophosphamide can damage the ovaries and cause premature menopause and permanent infertility. The risk of infertility in women increases with age and with the total dose of cyclophosphamide.

Rare: Scarring of the lung, liver problems, and allergic reactions are rare.

Interactions with Other Drugs

Allopurinol (*Zyloprim*): There is an increased risk of bone marrow suppression when cyclophosphamide is combined with allopurinol.

Thiazide diuretics ("water pills"): This combination can increase bone marrow suppression.

Other immunosuppressants: All drugs that suppress the immune system increase the risk of side effects such as infection. The more the immune system is suppressed, the higher the risk. High doses of corticosteroids, alone or with other drugs such as cyclophosphamide, increase the risk of infection.

Live vaccines: Some vaccines are given as a weaker strain of a live virus. These vaccines are usually avoided in people taking drugs that can suppress the immune system.

Important Information

- Avoid becoming pregnant while you are taking cyclophosphamide.
- Do not take more than the prescribed dose.
- Regular monitoring of your blood count and urine is important.
- Avoid immunizations (except for influenza and pneumonia) unless discussed with your physician.
- Contact your doctor if you develop any serious or prolonged infection or fever.
- Contact your doctor if you develop any blood in your urine.

Common Dose Sizes
Tablet: 25 mg, 50 mg.

Usual Adult Doses
The dose of cyclophosphamide is adjusted according to how you respond and by the change in your white blood cell count. Cyclophosphamide is usually given in one of two ways:

1. As tablets taken every morning. The dose of cyclophosphamide is usually chosen according to how big you are and how sensitive you are to cyclophosphamide. The usual range is 1 to 3 mg per kg body weight. Many people take somewhere between 100 mg and 150 mg a day. As you stay on cyclophosphamide longer, your dose may need to be reduced because your blood count can drop as your bone marrow becomes more sensitive to cyclophosphamide.
2. As an IV injection once every four weeks. A single large dose of cyclophosphamide, often about 1 g, is dissolved in saline and injected into a vein slowly over an hour or two. Drugs to prevent vomiting are often given before and after the IV cyclophosphamide dose.

Comments
Cyclophosphamide is not a drug that we use lightly. It is used only for serious problems that threaten life or organ function, and in these situations it can be lifesaving. Serious side effects can be decreased by careful monitoring. If you have a rheumatic problem that requires cyclophosphamide, I believe you should be monitored regularly by a rheumatologist.

The monthly IV way of taking cyclophosphamide is attractive because it may cause fewer side effects and causes very few bladder problems. The disadvantage is that you have to go to a doctor's office or hospital once a month, have an IV put in, and sit around while the drug is injected. Monthly IV doses are effective in systemic lupus erythematosus and are often used to treat serious lupus problems. In patients with vasculitis, such as Wegener's granulomatosis, monthly IV cyclophosphamide may not be as effective as daily oral cyclophosphamide, but this is controversial.

Mesna (see MESNA) is a drug that is sometimes used with the IV injections of cyclophosphamide to protect the bladder. Bladder problems are unusual with monthly IV cyclophosphamide, so some rheumatologists do not give Mesna.

CYCLOSPORINE

Brand Names

Sandimmune, Neoral.

Both of these preparations contain the identical drug—cyclosporine—but they are slightly different. *Neoral* is a newer preparation that is better absorbed than *Sandimmune.*

Sometimes Called

Cyclosporin, Cyclosporin A.

Drug Family

Cyclosporine is an antirejection drug that is used after organ transplantation. It changes the immune response and acts as a disease-modifying autirheumatic (DMARD) in RA.

Families of Arthritis Problems Prescribed For

Cyclosporine acts as a DMARD in RA. It is sometimes also tried for other problems, such as psoriasis and psoriatic arthritis, that are not responding to more standard treatments. Cyclosporine has been tried for just about every serious rheumatic problem not responding to other treatments, and there are reports of a few people responding to it. Examples of problems that have sometimes responded to cyclosporine are dermatomyositis, Behçet's disease (an uncommon problem that can cause mouth and genital ulcers and eye and joint problems), systemic lupus erythematosus, and eye problems occurring with other connective tissue problems.

How It Works

Cyclosporine has many effects, but an important one is that it decreases the production of a cytokine (chemical messenger) called interleukin–2 (or IL–2) by white blood cells; this and other effects suppress the immune response.

Avoid

Do not take cyclosporine if you are allergic to it. Cyclosporine is generally avoided in people who have poor kidney function, people who have had cancer, and in pregnancy.

Take Precautions

- Caution is needed in people with high blood pressure. The high blood pressure should be controlled before cyclosporine is started.
- You should keep out of the direct sun to minimize the risk of skin cancer.
- You will need regular monitoring of your blood while you are taking cyclosporine. The blood test that is usually checked is the creatinine level, a test of your kidney function. To protect against kidney problems, the dose of cyclosporine is decreased if your creatinine increases by more than 30 percent. This is a small increase and is usually still in the normal range for creatinine levels. This small increase is used to judge how sensitive your kidneys are to cyclosporine.
- Your blood pressure may increase on cyclosporine and needs to be checked from time to time.

• Good dental hygiene (brushing, flossing, and dental cleaning) will prevent cyclosporine from increasing gum growth.

Side Effects

Common: Stomach problems such as nausea, vomiting, gas, cramps, and diarrhea, which are unpleasant but not serious, are fairly common. Blood pressure can increase, usually only by a small amount, but in some people it will mean that they now need treatment for high blood pressure. A 30 percent or greater increase in your blood creatinine level is common and is used as a signal to decrease the dose. You may notice increased hair growth, usually fine downy hairs on the face and arms. Cyclosporine can increase the potassium and uric acid levels and lower the magnesium levels in your blood.

Less common: Shakiness (tremors), headache, muscle cramps, increased growth of the gums, and gout are less common.

Rare: Seizures, muscle, pancreas and liver problems, infection, and allergic reactions.

Interactions with Other Drugs

Many drugs interact with cyclosporine to increase or decrease its blood levels. With the low doses of cyclosporine used to treat rheumatic problems, these drug interactions are not usually a big problem and can usually be taken care of by adjusting the dose of cyclosporine if the interacting drug cannot be avoided.

Drugs that can increase the levels of cyclosporine.

Antifungal drugs such as ketoconazole (*Nizoral*), fluconazole (*Diflucan*), itraconazole (*Sporanox*), and miconazole injection (*Monistat*).

Some antibiotics such as erythromycin (*E.E.S, Erythrocin,* and many others), clarithromycin (*Biaxin*), and troландeomycin (*TAO*).

Some drugs used to treat HIV infection such as indinavir (*Crixivan*) and ritonavir (*Norvir*).

Some calcium channel blockers (a group of drugs used to treat high blood pressure, angina and Raynaud's): diltiazem (*Cardizem*), verapamil (*Calan, Isoptin*), and amlodipine (*Norvasc*).

Other drugs: allopurinol (*Zyloprim*), amiodarone (*Cordarone*), cimetidine (*Tagamet*), and grapefruit juice.

Drugs that can decrease the levels of cyclosporine.

Rifampin (*Rifadin, Rimactane*), phenytoin (*Dilantin*), phenobarbitone (*Barbita*), St. John's wort, and nafcillin (*Nafcil*).

Drugs that have an increased risk of side effects when combined with cyclosporine.

Diuretics such as amiloride (*Midamor*) and spironolactone (*Aldactone*) that hold onto potassium: Cyclosporine also causes your body to retain potassium, so the combination of these medicines increases the risk of a high potassium level in your blood.

Some drugs used to lower cholesterol: Lovastatin (*Mevacor*) and some of the other "statin" drugs can cause muscle damage. The risk of this is increased when these drugs are combined with cyclosporine.

Drugs that may be toxic to the kidneys: Aminoglycoside antibiotics, such as gentamicin (*Garamycin*), are more likely to increase the creatinine when they are combined with cyclosporine.

NSAIDs: Cyclosporine and NSAIDs are often combined, particularly in people with RA, but some experts try to avoid this combination if possible, particularly in people whose kidneys are sensitive to cyclosporine.

Others: Cyclosporine increases the blood levels of digoxin (*Lanoxin*).

Important Information

- Avoid becoming pregnant while you are taking cyclosporine.
- Do not take more than the prescribed dose of cyclosporine.
- Regular monitoring of your blood pressure and creatinine is important.
- Cyclosporine does not work very fast in RA and it may be eight to twelve weeks before you see a response.
- Cyclosporine interacts with many drugs. Make sure your physicians know that you are taking cyclosporine, and keep a copy of the cyclosporine package insert with you so that you can look up whether any new drug prescribed for you interacts with cyclosporine.

Common Dose Sizes

Capsule: 25 mg, 100 mg.

Usual Adult Doses

The starting dose for problems such as RA is 2.5 mg per kg body weight per day. The dose is usually split into two. So someone weighing 60 kg might be started on a cyclosporine dose of 75 mg twice a day. In overweight people the dose is usually calculated according to ideal weight, not actual weight. Your doctor may increase the dose slowly if you do not respond, and may decrease the dose if you have side effects. The maximum dose of cyclosporine for rheumatic problems is 4 mg per kg body weight a day for the *Neoral* preparation and 5 mg per kg body weight a day with the *Sandimmune* preparation. The average effective dose of cyclosporine in RA is about 3 mg per kg a day. Going above 5 mg per kg a day increases the risks of side effects. The dose of the two preparations available (*Neoral* and *Sandimmune*) is similar, but often when people switch from *Sandimmune* to the better absorbed *Neoral,* they can decrease their dose by about a quarter.

Comments

Cyclosporine is a relatively new drug for treating RA. It is effective, but it is no more effective than other DMARDs. Because it is expensive and needs careful monitoring, it is often reserved as a DMARD for people who cannot take or do not respond to other DMARDs. Cyclosporine is also effective in combination treatments—combined with methotrexate or with hydroxychloroquine. For people who have had an incomplete response to treatment with a single DMARD, these combinations are more effective than the single drugs. Cyclosporine is reasonably well tolerated, and in clinical trials most people have been able to continue taking it for a year. But with treatment for two years or longer, some people have a small increase in their creatinine that does not come back down when their dose of cyclosporine is decreased, and they have to stop taking it. There is little long-term information about the methotrexate plus cyclosporine combination treatment in RA. But there is a lot of safety information from many thousands of people who have had organ transplants and have taken cyclosporine, often in combination with prednisone and azathioprine, for many years.

Cyclosporine blood levels are often measured in people who have had organ transplants, and their dose of cyclosporine is adjusted to prevent the transplant from being rejected. In people with rheumatic problems, cyclosporine blood levels are seldom measured because the blood levels do not predict how you will respond.

CYTOTEC (SEE MISOPROSTOL)

CYTOXAN (SEE CYCLOPHOSPHAMIDE)

DANAZOL

Brand Name

Danocrine.

Drug Family

Danazol suppresses the release of hormones from the pituitary gland.

Families of Arthritis Problems Prescribed For

Danazol is not used to treat arthritis itself. It is used to treat some uncommon problems that can be arthritis-related. For example, it is sometimes used to increase the platelet count in people who have low platelets caused by a problem such as lupus. Danazol is also used to prevent attacks of a problem called hereditary angioedema, which causes swelling of the tongue, lips, and mouth. More often danazol is used to treat endometriosis and fibrocystic breast disease in women who do not have arthritis problems.

How It Works

Danazol, a mild androgen (male hormone), is thought to prevent attacks of angioedema by increasing the blood levels of a substance called complement.

Avoid

Do not take danazol if you are allergic to it. Danazol is avoided in pregnancy and in people with liver or kidney problems.

Take Precautions

- If you have vaginal bleeding and the cause is not known, this must be evaluated before you start danazol.
- Caution is needed if danazol is used in people who have had blood clots in their veins (deep vein thrombosis) or who have had strokes or blood clots in other places (emboli).

Side Effects

Common: Side effects caused by the male hormone (androgenic) effects of danazol are acne, increased facial and body hair, irregular menstrual cycles, bleeding between monthly cycles, weight gain, and fluid retention. Abnormal liver function tests are common.

Rare: Uncommon problems are jaundice or serious liver problems, inflammation of the pancreas, a low platelet or white blood cell count, rashes and headache caused by increased pressure inside the brain.

Interactions with Other Drugs

Warfarin (*Coumadin*): Danazol can increase the anticoagulant (anti–blood clotting) effect of warfarin in some people. If you are taking warfarin to prevent blood clots and you start taking danazol, you may need to have your blood monitored more frequently than usual, and your dose of warfarin may need to be changed.

Carbamazepine (*Tegretol*): Danazol can increase carbamazepine concentrations.

Important Information

• Make sure you are not pregnant before you start danazol, and use a nonhormonal contraceptive to prevent pregnancy.

• Keep out of the direct sun. Danazol can make your skin more sensitive to the sun.

Common Dose Sizes

Capsules: 50 mg, 100 mg, 200 mg.

Usual Adult Doses

For hereditary angioedema the usual adult dose of danazol is 400 to 600 mg a day, divided into two or three doses.

Comments

Danazol is an unusual drug that is used for uncommon arthritis-related problems.

DANOCRINE (SEE DANAZOL)

DAPSONE

Brand Names

Avlosulfon.

Drug Family

Dapsone is related to the sulfonamide (sulfa) antibiotics.

Families of Arthritis Problems Prescribed For

Dapsone was tried for RA and is modestly effective, but it has been replaced by safer and more effective treatments. Dapsone is used for other arthritis-related problems, but even then it is usually tried only after other treatments have not worked. It is sometimes tried in people who have a bad skin rash caused by systemic or discoid lupus erythematosus. It is also sometimes used for vasculitis that affects mainly the skin and for an uncommon ulcerating rash called pyoderma gangrenosum.

How It Works

We do not know for certain how dapsone works, but it may alter white blood cell function.

Avoid

Do not take dapsone if you are allergic to it or if you are pregnant.

Take Precautions

- Caution is needed in people who are allergic to sulfonamides ("sulfa" drugs).
- People who have inherited low levels of an enzyme called glucose-6 phosphate dehydrogenase (G-6PD) can break down their red blood cells when they take dapsone. G-6PD deficiency is more common in certain ethnic groups (African, Mediterranean, East Asian). In people belonging to these ethnic groups, a blood test to check for G-6PD deficiency is often done before treatment with dapsone is started.
- Your blood count will be monitored frequently, particularly when you begin treatment. Liver tests are usually checked from time to time.

Side Effects

Common: Dapsone can lead to the breakdown of red blood cells, called hemolysis, and cause anemia—even in people who are not G-6PD deficient. This side effect increases with the dose of dapsone. Dapsone can also increase the blood concentrations of a type of hemoglobin that does not carry oxygen very well, called methemoglobin, and this can cause people to look a purplish color. A rash and GI symptoms are fairly common.

Rare: A very low white blood cell count, a serious peeling skin rash, and serious liver problems are rare.

Interaction with Other Drugs

Rifampin (*Rimactane*): Treatment with rifampin can decrease the blood levels of dapsone.

Drugs that block the effects of folic acid, such as trimethoprim and sulfonamide antibiotics (*Bactrim* and many others): These can increase the side effects of dapsone.

Important Information

• Make sure that you have the recommended blood tests done.

Common Dose Sizes

Tablets: 25 mg, 100 mg.

Usual Adult Doses

The usual adult starting dose of dapsone is 50 mg a day. This is increased, if needed, up to 100 mg a day. Some people tolerate doses higher than 100 mg a day, but side effects are more common.

Comments

Dapsone is not the drug of first choice for any rheumatic problem, but in a few people who don't respond to other treatments it can sometimes be useful. Side effects are common and limit its use.

DARVOCET (SEE ACETAMINOPHEN + NARCOTICS)

DARVON (SEE PROPOXYPHENE)

DAYPRO (SEE OXAPROZIN)

DEMEROL (SEE MEPERIDINE)

DEPEN (SEE PENICILLAMINE)

DEPOMEDROL (SEE CORTICOSTEROIDS, INTRA-ARTICULAR)

DESYREL (TRAZODONE; SEE *PROFILES OF COMMON ANTIDEPRESSANT DRUGS* UNDER AMITRIPTYLINE)

DEXAMETHASONE (SEE CORTICOSTEROIDS)

DHEA

DHEA is not approved by the FDA for the treatment or prevention of any medical problem, but it is available in health-food stores.

Sometimes Called

Dehdroepiandrosterone.

Drug Family

DHEA is a steroid that is made by your adrenal glands. It is a precursor (building block) that is converted into both male (testosterone) and female (estrone, estradiol) hormones.

Families of Arthritis Problems Prescribed For

DHEA has received a lot of publicity as a treatment for systemic lupus erythematosus (SLE) and as an antiaging hormone.

How It Works

DHEA was tried in SLE because many people with lupus have low DHEA levels and because DHEA was effective in animal models of lupus. DHEA is a precursor (building block) that is used to make many male and female hormones.

Comments

In a few clinical trials, DHEA has improved the symptoms of depression and has stabilized bone density in people with osteoporosis. The effects of DHEA in lupus clinical trials have been mildly positive but unimpressive. Many people don't realize that DHEA acts as a hormone and that it increases the formation of other hormones, particularly male hormones. Androgenic (male hormone type) side effects such as acne, greasy hair, changed menstrual patterns, and increased body hair, are mild but common. DHEA has definite effects. It is acting as a drug, and it should be tested like any other drug. Until more high-quality information is available about how safe and how effective DHEA is, I would not recommend it for any arthritis-related problem. We know that male and female hormones can have strong effects, both good and bad, on many medical problems, particularly some cancers. We need good information about the long-term effects of any hormone treatment, including DHEA, to know how safe and effective it is.

DICLOFENAC

Brand Names

Cataflam (immediate-release), *Voltaren* (enteric-coated, extended-release), *Arthrotec* (diclofenac + misoprostol)

Drug Family

Diclofenac belongs to the nonsteroidal anti-inflammatory drug (NSAID) family. There are two big groups of NSAIDs, divided by whether they inhibit both cyclo-oxygenase (COX) enzymes, COX-1 and COX-2, or are more selective for COX-2. Diclofenac inhibits both COX-1 and COX-2. *Arthrotec* combines an NSAID (Diclofenac) with misoprostol, a drug that protects against peptic ulcers.

Families of Arthritis Problems Prescribed For

NSAIDs are used to treat all kinds of pain and inflammation, whether they affect the joints or not. NSAIDs are used to treat many kinds of arthritis problems, such as RA, osteoarthritis, rheumatic fever, Still's disease (also known as juvenile rheumatoid arthritis), gout, ankylosing spondylitis, and bursitis. NSAIDs decrease pain and inflammation, but they do not change the progression of arthritis.

How It Works

Most NSAIDs inhibit the enzymes COX-1 and COX-2. Inhibiting these cyclo-oxygenase enzymes decreases the formation of chemicals called prostaglandins. Decreasing the prostaglandins made by COX-2 is anti-inflammatory, which is usually why we use NSAIDs. Inhibiting COX-1 makes platelets in your blood less sticky, which is why aspirin is used to prevent heart attacks. COX-1 also protects the stomach from ulcers, and blocking COX-1 may be why the risk of peptic ulcers is increased with many NSAIDs.

Arthrotec combines the NSAID diclofenac with the GI-protective drug misoprostol to decrease the risk of peptic ulcers caused by the NSAID.

Avoid

Do not take diclofenac if you are allergic to it. People who have had a serious allergic reaction (swelling of the face and tongue, and wheezing) to one NSAID can have the same reaction to others. People with asthma or nasal polyps are more likely to be allergic to NSAIDs.

NSAIDs are avoided if someone has an active peptic ulcer, is bleeding, or is pregnant.

The misoprostol component of *Arthrotec* can cause abortion and abnormalities in the unborn baby and should be avoided in pregnancy.

Take Precautions

- NSAIDs can cause fluid retention and can worsen heart failure and high blood pressure.
- Some people have a higher risk for peptic ulcers caused by NSAIDs. Risk factors are being older than 65 years, having had a previous peptic ulcer, having had a previous bleeding ulcer, and taking a corticosteroid. In people who have a higher risk for peptic ulcers caused by NSAIDs, most rheumatologists would avoid NSAIDs if possible. If this is not possible, then prescribing misoprostol (see MISOPROSTOL—*Cytotec*) or a proton pump inhibitor (see OMEPRAZOLE—*Prilosec*) to protect against peptic ulcers caused by NSAIDs is an option. Another option is to use a COX-2 selective NSAID (see CELECOXIB—*Celebrex* and ROFECOXIB—*Vioxx*). *Arthrotec* combines diclofenac and misoprostol. None of these choices is foolproof, and peptic ulcers can still happen.

• NSAIDs have to be used carefully in people who have asthma, a bleeding problem, or liver or kidney problems.

• If you are taking NSAIDs regularly, blood tests will be done from time to time to check your blood count (in case you are losing blood slowly from an ulcer that you may not know about), your creatinine (for kidney function), and liver enzymes. People taking diuretics ("water pills") or ACE (angiotensin converting enzyme) inhibitors—a family of drugs that lower blood pressure—and people with diabetes, heart failure, or existing kidney problems are more likely to have kidney problems caused by NSAIDs. These people may need more frequent blood tests to check their kidney function.

• If you are a woman who could become pregnant, pregnancy must be ruled out before you start treatment with misoprostol or *Arthrotec.* You must use reliable contraception while you are taking misoprostol or *Arthrotec.* I find it more convenient to avoid misoprostol in women who could become pregnant and to use an alternative strategy for GI protection.

Side Effects

For the side effects of the misoprostol component of *Arthrotec,* see MISOPROSTOL. For the side effects of diclofenac, see NSAIDs.

Interaction with Other Drugs

See NSAIDs.

Important Information

• Taking NSAIDs with food is a good idea and may protect you from indigestion, but it does not prevent peptic ulcers.

• To minimize your GI risks, use the lowest effective dose of an NSAID.

• One of the signs that you may be bleeding from the stomach is if you have pitch-black bowel movements. Bowel movements with altered blood, in addition to being black, are also often runny and very smelly. If this happens, contact your doctor immediately.

Common Dose Sizes

Tablet: Diclofenac 25 mg, 50 mg, 75 mg, 100 mg extended-release; Diclofenac 50 mg + Misoprostol 200 micrograms (*Arthrotec 50*); Diclofenac 75 mg + Misoprostol 200 micrograms (*Arthrotec 75*).

Usual Adult Doses

Diclofenac: The usual adult dose is 150 to 200 mg a day divided into two to four doses.

Arthrotec 50: The usual adult dose is one tablet taken two or three times a day.

Arthrotec 75: The usual adult dose is one tablet taken twice a day.

Comments

See NSAIDs.

The fixed combination of an NSAID (diclofenac) and a GI-protecting drug (misoprostol), *Arthrotec,* is convenient for some people, but many people prefer to have their NSAID and their GI-protective drugs as separate tablets because it is more convenient if they need to adjust the dose of only one of the medicines.

DIDRONEL (SEE ETIDRONATE)

DIFLUNISAL

Brand Name

Dolobid.

Drug Family

Diflunisal is a nonsteroidal anti-inflammatory drug (NSAID). There are two big groups of NSAIDs, divided by whether they inhibit both cyclo-oxygenase (COX) enzymes, COX-1 and COX-2, or are more selective for COX-2. Diflunisal inhibits both COX-1 and COX-2.

Families of Arthritis Problems Prescribed For

NSAIDs are used to treat all kinds of pain and inflammation, whether they affect the joints or not. NSAIDs are used to treat many kinds of arthritis problems, such as RA, osteoarthritis, and bursitis. NSAIDs decrease pain and inflammation, but they do not change the progression of arthritis.

How It Works

Most NSAIDs inhibit the enzymes COX-1 and COX-2. Inhibiting these cyclo-oxygenase enzymes decreases the formation of chemicals called prostaglandins. Decreasing the prostaglandins made by COX-2 is anti-inflammatory, which is usually why we use NSAIDs. Inhibiting COX-1 makes platelets in your blood less sticky, which is why aspirin is used to prevent heart attacks. COX-1 also protects the stomach from ulcers, and blocking COX-1 may be why the risk of peptic ulcers is increased with many NSAIDs.

Avoid

Do not take diflunisal if you are allergic to it. People who have had a serious allergic reaction (swelling of the face and tongue, and wheezing) to one NSAID can have the same reaction with others. People with asthma or nasal polyps are more likely to be allergic to NSAIDs. NSAIDs are avoided if someone has an active peptic ulcer, is bleeding, or is pregnant.

Take Precautions

• NSAIDs can cause fluid retention and can worsen heart failure and high blood pressure.

• Some people have a higher risk for peptic ulcers caused by NSAIDs. Risk factors are being older than 65 years, having had a previous peptic ulcer, having had a previous bleeding ulcer, and taking a corticosteroid. In people at higher risk for peptic ulcers caused by NSAIDs, most rheumatologists would avoid an NSAID, if possible. If this is not possible, then prescribing misoprostol (see MISOPROSTOL—*Cytotec*) or a proton pump inhibitor (see OMEPRAZOLE—*Prilosec*) to protect against peptic ulcers caused by NSAIDs is an option. Another option is to use a COX-2 selective NSAID (see CELECOXIB—*Celebrex* and ROFECOXIB—*Vioxx*). None of these choices is foolproof, and peptic ulcers can still happen.

• NSAIDs have to be used carefully in people who have asthma, a bleeding problem, or liver or kidney problems.

• If you are taking NSAIDs regularly, blood tests will be done from time to time to check your blood count (in case you are losing blood slowly from an ulcer that you may not know about), your creatinine (for kidney function), and liver enzymes. People taking diuretics ("water pills") or ACE (angiotensin converting enzyme) inhibitors—a family of drugs that lowers blood pressure—and people with diabetes, heart failure, or existing kidney problems are more likely to have kidney problems caused by NSAIDs. These people may need more frequent blood tests to check their kidney function.

Side Effects

See NSAIDs.

Interactions with Other Drugs

See NSAIDs.

Important Information

- Taking NSAIDs with food is a good idea and may protect you from indigestion, but it does not prevent peptic ulcers.
- To minimize your GI risks, use the lowest effective dose of an NSAID.
- One of the signs that you may be bleeding from the stomach is if you have pitch-black bowel movements. Bowel movements with altered blood, in addition to being black, are also often runny and very smelly. If this happens, contact your doctor immediately.

Common Dose Sizes

Tablet: 250 mg, 500 mg.

Usual Adult Doses

The usual adult dose of diflunisal is 500 mg to 1,000 mg a day, divided into two doses.

Comments

See NSAIDs.

DISALCID (SEE SALSALATE)

DOLOBID (SEE DIFLUNISAL)

DOXEPIN (*SINEQUAN*; SEE ***PROFILES OF COMMON ANTIDEPRESSANT DRUGS*** UNDER AMITRIPTYLINE)

DOXYCYCLINE (SEE TETRACYCLINE)

DURAGESIC (SEE FENTANYL)

EASPRIN (SEE ASPIRIN)

ECOTRIN (SEE ASPIRIN)

ELAVIL (SEE AMITRIPTYLINE)

ENBREL (SEE ETANERCEPT)

ETANERCEPT

Brand Name
Enbrel.

Sometimes Called
TNF (tumor necrosis factor) antagonist.

Drug Family
Etanercept acts as a disease-modifying antirheumatic drug (DMARD) in RA.

Families of Arthritis Problems Prescribed For

Etanercept is used to treat rheumatoid arthritis and juvenile rheumatoid arthritis. There are a few reports about it being used for vasculitis, but the information is very preliminary.

How It Works

Etanercept is a biological drug; it is a protein specially designed to block the effects of tumor necrosis factor (TNF), a cytokine (chemical messenger) that your body makes and that is responsible for some of the inflammation in RA. To cause inflammation, TNF has to bind onto special TNF receptors that are found in various tissues in your body. Etanercept consists of two receptors for TNF joined together. The TNF that your body makes binds to the "false" etanercept receptors and not the "real" receptors. In other words, etanercept mops up the TNF your body makes before it gets to the real receptors, where it would activate inflammation.

Avoid

Do not take etanercept if you are allergic to it or have an active infection. Etanercept is usually avoided in people who have had cancer, particularly lymphoma.

Take Precautions

- Etanercept may suppress your immune response; take any infections seriously and have them treated early.
- If you develop a serious infection, stop etanercept and contact your doctor.
- Caution is advised in people with multiple sclerosis (MS) or optic neuritis.

Side Effects

Etanercept, so far, is remarkably safe.

Common: Minor skin reactions, with redness and itching around the injection site, are common but seldom a problem.

Rare: Infections, some serious, have occurred, but at this stage it is not clear if etanercept increases the risks of infection, and if it does, by how much. There is no evidence that the risk of cancer is increased in people who have taken etanercept, but it will be several years before we have enough information about this. Some people, about 5 to 10 percent of those using etanercept, will develop a positive antinuclear antibody (ANA) test. The ANA is a blood test that is positive in people with lupus but is also positive in many healthy people. So there is the worry that etanercept may increase the risk of autoimmune problems such as lupus. So far this has not been a problem. Bone marrow suppression resulting in low blood cell counts and neurological problems similar to multiple sclerosis have occurred with anti-TNF drugs, but they are very rare.

Interactions with Other Drugs

Vaccines: Live virus vaccines are avoided in people taking etanercept.

Important Information

- Avoid becoming pregnant while you are taking etanercept.
- Avoid immunizations (except for influenza and pneumonia) unless discussed with your physician.
- Contact your doctor if you develop any serious or prolonged infection or fever.
- Etanercept should be stored in the refrigerator.

Common Dose Sizes

Etanercept comes as a vial that contains 25 mg—enough for one injection.

Usual Adult Doses

The usual adult dose of etanercept is 25 mg injected under the skin of your thigh, arm, or abdomen twice a week.

Comments

Etanercept was the first biological drug approved for treating RA, and it is likely to become one of the most widely used biological agents. It is extremely effective and, so far, very safe.

Etanercept is about as effective as methotrexate. About 40 percent of people who got etanercept in clinical trials had a 50 percent or greater response in their overall RA activity. These are very impressive results and, considering efficacy, put etanercept up at or near the top of the DMARD pile. People respond very quickly to anti-TNF drugs, unlike other DMARDs, and they often feel better within a couple of weeks. But like all DMARDs, not everyone responds to anti-TNF treatment. Clinical studies have shown that people who are not well controlled on etanercept alone do better when etanercept is combined with methotrexate.

There are a couple of drawbacks.

1. It has to be given by injection. Most people don't consider this a problem. The injections are given under the skin, just like insulin injections in people with diabetes, and it is not a big deal.
2. Etanercept is very expensive, costing at least ten times more than most traditional DMARD treatments. On the other hand, poorly controlled RA can be very expensive if one thinks of things such as decreased income, a poor quality of life, and joint-replacement surgery.
3. We are accumulating long-term information about side effects. At the moment TNF blockers seem to be unusu-

ally safe drugs, but we will know the answers to the really important questions—such as the risks of cancer—only in a few years time.

Anti-TNF drugs are a huge advance in the treatment of RA, but they are not for everyone. If you have mild or moderate RA that is well controlled with standard DMARDs, there is no advantage to switching to an anti-TNF drug. On the other hand, if you have RA that remains active in spite of standard DMARD treatment or combination DMARD treatment, and if your health insurance covers anti-TNF treatment or you can afford it, this treatment could be for you.

There are two anti-TNF drugs on the market, etanercept (*Enbrel*) and Infliximab (*Remicade*). They work in different ways and are given differently. Etanercept is given by an injection under the skin twice a week, and infliximab is given as an intravenous infusion at zero, two and six weeks and then every eight weeks. It is standard practice to combine infliximab with methotrexate, mainly to suppress antibodies that your body could make against the drug. This is not the case with etanercept, which can be used alone, without methotrexate.

ETIDRONATE

Brand Name

Didronel.

Sometimes Called

Disodium Etidronate, Sodium Etidronate.

Drug Family

Etidronate belongs to the family of drugs that prevents bone loss. Is a bisphosphonate.

Families of Arthritis Problems Prescribed For

Etidronate is used to treat and prevent osteoporosis. Remember that osteoporosis means "thin bones" and is not a type of arthritis. The aim of treatment is to prevent fractures. Etidronate is also sometimes used to treat Paget's disease.

How It Works

Bone is continually replaced as it is resorbed, and then new bone is laid down. Etidronate slows down the resorption of bone but does not increase bone formation. Etidronate will stabilize or slightly increase bone density.

Avoid

Do not take etidronate if you are allergic to it.

Take Precautions

Caution is needed in people who have poor kidney function, and the dose may need to be decreased. If the bone problems of Paget's disease have resorbed a lot of bone and there is a risk that these bones may break, etidronate is not usually used.

Side Effects

Common: Nausea, diarrhea, and a metallic taste can occur, but most people tolerate etidronate well, and GI problems are less common than with alendronate.

Rare: An allergic rash, fever, bone pain, and a low blood calcium level are uncommon.

Interactions with Other Drugs

Any drug: Etidronate is poorly absorbed, and if you take it at the same time as any other drug, or even with food, it may not be absorbed.

Important Information

• Etidronate should be taken on an empty stomach with a full glass of water.

• Do not eat or drink anything, other than water, for at least thirty minutes after you have taken etidronate. Even coffee or fruit juice stops the etidronate from getting into your body. If you can wait an hour before eating or drinking something else, so much the better, because more etidronate will be absorbed into your body.

• Take etidronate by itself. Delay taking your other medicines for at least an hour.

Common Dose Sizes

Tablets: 200 mg, 400 mg.

Usual Adult Doses

For osteoporosis the usual adult dose of etidronate is 400 mg a day for fourteen days out of every three months. Calcium (1 g a day) and a vitamin D (400 IU a day) supplement are also usually taken. Etidronate stabilizes osteoporosis and does not cure it, so treatment needs to continue for a long time.

For Paget's disease the usual dose is 5 mg per kg of body weight a day for up to six months, but etidronate has largely been replaced by newer bisphosphonates for treating Paget's disease.

Comments

Osteoporosis is a common problem, particularly in women after the menopause and in people taking corticosteroids. Osteoporosis is diagnosed by measuring your bone density, often with a type of scan known as a DEXA (dual energy X-ray absorptiometry). The usual program for treating or preventing osteoporosis also includes stopping smoking and drinking alcohol, increasing exercise, taking calcium supplements and often a low dose of vitamin D.

Alendronate is the bisphosphonate that has the most supporting evidence to show that it actually decreases the risk of fracture. Etidronate is useful for some people who cannot take alendronate because they have problems swallowing or have bad esophageal reflux. Don't forget that the aim of treating osteoporosis is to prevent fractures and that many fractures are caused by falls. Simple things can reduce your risk of falling. Some of these may apply to you. Get rid of loose throw rugs and other objects that can trip you, have nonslip surfaces, use a cane if you need one, don't hurry—that telephone can keep ringing—and keep a night-light on so that you can see your way to the bathroom. People with poor vision are more likely to fall, so have your vision checked from time to time. Alcohol and medicines that affect your balance, such as many kinds of sleeping pills, increase your risk of falling. Avoid them if possible.

ETODOLAC

Brand Name

Lodine.

Drug Family

Etodolac is a nonsteroidal anti-inflammatory drug (NSAID). There are two big groups of NSAIDs, divided by whether they inhibit both cyclo-oxygenase (COX) enzymes, COX-1 and COX-2, or are more selective for COX-2. Etodolac inhibits both COX-1 and COX-2, and while not highly selective for COX-2, tends to have more COX-2 blocking effect than COX-1 blocking effect.

Families of Arthritis Problems Prescribed For

NSAIDs are used to treat all kinds of pain and inflammation, whether they affect the joints or not. NSAIDs are used to treat many kinds of arthritis problems, such as RA, osteoarthritis, and bursitis. NSAIDs decrease pain and inflammation, but they do not change the progression of arthritis.

How It Works

Most NSAIDs inhibit the enzymes COX-1 and COX-2. Inhibiting these cyclo-oxygenase enzymes decreases the formation of chemicals called prostaglandins. Decreasing the prostaglandins made by COX-2 is anti-inflammatory, which is usually why we use NSAIDs. Inhibiting COX-1 makes platelets in your blood less sticky, which is why aspirin is used to prevent heart attacks. COX-1 also protects the stomach from ulcers, and blocking COX-1 may be why the risk of peptic ulcers is increased with many NSAIDs. Because etodolac tends more toward a COX-2 blocking effect, it may be kinder on the stomach than nonselective NSAIDs.

Avoid

Do not take etodolac if you are allergic to it. People who have had a serious allergic reaction (swelling of the face and tongue, and wheezing) to one NSAID can have the same reaction to others. People with asthma or nasal polyps are more likely to be allergic to NSAIDs. NSAIDs are avoided if someone has an active peptic ulcer, is bleeding, or is pregnant.

Take Precautions

- NSAIDs can cause fluid retention and can worsen heart failure and high blood pressure.
- Some people have a higher risk for peptic ulcers caused by NSAIDs. Risk factors are being older than 65 years, having

had a previous peptic ulcer, having had a previous bleeding ulcer, and taking a corticosteroid. In people at higher risk for peptic ulcers caused by NSAIDs, most rheumatologists would avoid an NSAID, if possible. If this is not possible, prescribing misoprostol (see MISOPROSTOL—*Cytotec*) or a proton pump inhibitor (see OMEPRAZOLE—*Prilosec*) to protect against peptic ulcers caused by NSAIDs is an option. Another option is to use a COX-2 selective NSAID (see CELECOXIB—*Celebrex* and ROFECOXIB—*Vioxx*). None of these choices is foolproof, and peptic ulcers can still happen.

- NSAIDs have to be used carefully in people who have asthma, a bleeding problem, or liver or kidney problems.
- If you are taking NSAIDs regularly, blood tests will be done from time to time to check your blood count (in case you are losing blood slowly from an ulcer that you may not know about), your creatinine (for kidney function), and liver enzymes. People taking diuretics ("water pills") or ACE (angiotensin converting enzyme) inhibitors—a family of drugs that lowers blood pressure—and people with diabetes, heart failure, or existing kidney problems are more likely to have kidney problems caused by NSAIDs. These people may need more frequent blood tests to check their kidney function.

Side Effects

See NSAIDs.

Etodolac is one of the nonselective NSAIDs that causes fewer GI problems.

Interaction with Other Drugs

See NSAIDs.

Important Information

• Taking NSAIDs with food is a good idea and may protect you from indigestion, but it does not prevent peptic ulcers.

• To minimize your GI risks, use the lowest effective dose of an NSAID.

• One of the signs that you may be bleeding from the stomach is if you have pitch-black bowel movements. Bowel movements with altered blood, in addition to being black, are also often runny and very smelly. If this happens, contact your doctor immediately.

Common Dose Sizes

Capsule: 200 mg, 300 mg.
Tablet: 400 mg.

Usual Adult Doses

The usual adult dose of etodolac is 200 to 400 mg taken two or three times a day. The maximum daily dose is 1,000 mg.

Comments.

See NSAIDs.

There is some information showing that etodolac may cause fewer GI problems than other commonly used nonselective NSAIDs.

EVISTA (SEE RALOXIFENE)

FAMOTIDINE (*PEPCID*; SEE ***PROFILES OF COMMON*** H_2***-RECEPTOR ANTAGONIST DRUGS*** UNDER CIMETIDINE)

FELDENE (SEE PIROXICAM)

FENOPROFEN

Brand Name
Nalfon.

Other Names
Fenoprofen calcium.

Drug Family
Fenoprofen is a nonsteroidal anti-inflammatory drug (NSAID). There are two big groups of NSAIDs, divided by whether they inhibit both cyclo-oxygenase (COX) enzymes, COX-1 and COX-2, or are more selective for COX-2. Fenoprofen inhibits both COX-1 and COX-2.

Families of Arthritis Problems Prescribed For
NSAIDs are used to treat all kinds of pain and inflammation, whether they affect the joints or not. NSAIDs are used to treat many kinds of arthritis problems, such as RA, osteoarthritis, and bursitis. NSAIDs decrease pain and inflammation, but they do not change the progression of arthritis.

How It Works
Most NSAIDs inhibit the enzymes COX-1 and COX-2. Inhibiting these cyclo-oxygenase enzymes decreases the formation of chemicals called prostaglandins. Decreasing the prostaglandins made by COX-2 is anti-inflammatory, which is usually why we use NSAIDs. Inhibiting COX-1 makes platelets in your blood less sticky, which is why aspirin is used to treat heart attacks. COX-1 also protects the stomach from ulcers, and blocking COX-1 may be why the risk of peptic ulcers is increased with many NSAIDs.

Avoid

Do not take fenoprofen if you are allergic to it. People who have had a serious allergic reaction (swelling of the face and tongue, and wheezing) to one NSAID can have the same reaction with others. People with asthma or nasal polyps are more likely to be allergic to NSAIDs. NSAIDs are avoided if someone has an active peptic ulcer, is bleeding, or is pregnant.

Take Precautions

• NSAIDs can cause fluid retention and can worsen heart failure and high blood pressure.

• Some people have a higher risk for peptic ulcers caused by NSAIDs. Risk factors are being older than 65 years, having had a previous peptic ulcer, having had a previous bleeding ulcer, and taking a corticosteroid. In people at higher risk for peptic ulcers caused by NSAIDs, most rheumatologists would avoid an NSAID, if possible. If this is not possible, then prescribing misoprostol (see MISOPROSTOL—*Cytotec*) or a proton pump inhibitor (see OMEPRAZOLE—*Prilosec*) to protect against peptic ulcers caused by NSAIDs is an option. Another option is to use a COX-2 selective NSAID (see CELECOXIB—*Celebrex* and ROFECOXIB—*Vioxx*). None of these choices is foolproof, and peptic ulcers can still happen.

• NSAIDs have to be used carefully in people who have asthma, a bleeding problem, or liver or kidney problems.

• If you are taking NSAIDs regularly, blood tests will be done from time to time to check your blood count (in case you are losing blood slowly from an ulcer that you may not know about), your creatinine (for kidney function), and liver enzymes. People taking diuretics ("water pills") or ACE (angiotensin converting enzyme) inhibitors—a family of drugs that lowers blood pressure—and people with diabetes, heart failure, or existing kidney problems are more likely to have kidney problems caused by NSAIDs. These people may need more frequent blood tests to check their kidney function.

Side Effects

See NSAIDs.

Interactions with Other Drugs

See NSAIDs.

Important Information

- Taking NSAIDs with food is a good idea and may protect you from indigestion, but it does not prevent peptic ulcers.
- To minimize your GI risks, use the lowest effective dose of an NSAID.
- One of the signs that you may be bleeding from the stomach is if you have pitch-black bowel movements. Bowel movements with altered blood, in addition to being black, are also often runny and very smelly. If this happens, contact your doctor immediately.

Common Dose Sizes

Capsule: 200 mg, 300 mg; Tablet: 600 mg.

Usual Adult Doses

The usual adult dose of fenoprofen is 300 to 600 mg taken three or four times a day.

Comments

See NSAIDs.

FENTANYL

Brand Names

Duragesic, Sublimaze.

Drug Family

Fentanyl is a strong narcotic analgesic (painkiller).

Families of Arthritis Problems Prescribed For

Fentanyl is used for severe uncontrolled pain. Strong narcotic analgesics are usually prescribed only for pain that is not controlled by acetaminophen alone or an NSAID alone or by weaker narcotics, such as codeine or hydrocodone. Narcotics do not affect inflammation.

How It Works

Narcotics decrease pain by acting through specific receptors in the brain.

Avoid

Do not use fentanyl if you are allergic to it. Real allergic reactions are rare, but a lot of people get side effects, such as nausea or feeling "spacy," from narcotics. Avoid fentanyl if you have had an addiction problem.

Take Precautions

- Don't drink alcohol while you are taking narcotics.
- There is a risk of becoming addicted to narcotics. Use narcotics only for pain, not to feel good. If possible, limit the dose and how long you take them. One physician should be responsible for all your narcotic prescriptions so that everyone knows what painkillers you are taking.
- Caution is needed in older people and in people with liver, lung, or kidney problems.

Side Effects

The side effects of strong narcotics are common but usually mild. People vary in their sensitivity to different narcotics.

Common: Nausea, vomiting, constipation, poor appetite,

dizziness, lightheadedness or feeling "spacy," sleepiness, low blood pressure, and a slow heart rate are common.

Less common: An allergic reaction with rash, hives, or asthma is less common. Confusion, feeling nervous or agitated, sleeping badly, feeling "high," becoming addicted and trying to get higher doses of narcotic to feel good rather than to control pain can occur. Too high a dose of fentanyl suppresses the drive to breathe.

Interactions with Other Drugs

Any other sedative drug: Narcotics make people sleepy, and an overdose can make people unconscious. Combining a narcotic with another sedative drug, such as alcohol, is dangerous.

Monoamine oxidase inhibitor (MAOI) antidepressants: There is an increased risk of a hypertensive crisis (dangerously high blood pressure and severe heart problems) if fentanyl and MAOI drugs are combined.

Important Information

- Don't take more than the prescribed dose.
- Don't drink alcohol while you are taking narcotic painkillers.
- Narcotics can cause drowsiness and affect your concentration when driving and performing other tasks.
- Fentanyl is a narcotic and can be addictive (see Comments).
- Narcotics are dangerous in overdose and must be kept away from children.

Common Dose Sizes

There is a fentanyl injection that is used as an anesthetic drug, but the way fentanyl is most often prescribed for pain is as a patch (transdermal preparation). This comes in different sizes that release different amounts of fentanyl per hour.

Transdermal system: 25 micrograms per hour, 50 micrograms per hour, 75 micrograms per hour, and 100 micrograms per hour.

Usual Adult Doses

For pain control in adults, the usual starting dose of fentanyl is the 25 micogram per hour patch. This can be increased if needed. In most people the patch is changed every seventy-two hours. The patch needs to be applied to dry, nonhairy skin on the trunk or upper arms.

Comments

Fentanyl can suppress the drive to breathe for longer than it suppresses pain. There is a danger, particularly in older people or people with lung problems, of suppressing the drive to breathe with high doses of fentanyl. The absorption of fentanyl from the patch can be increased if you have a fever. The fentanyl patch is convenient for long-term control of continuous pain, but because it starts to work so slowly, it is not useful for controlling pain immediately. If a new dose is started, the effects on pain can be evaluated after twenty-four hours.

There is some controversy about how narcotic analgesics should be used to control chronic "benign" pain, meaning chronic pain not caused by cancer. This is particularly true of the strong narcotics such as morphine and fentanyl. Some physicians think that the risk of addiction and abuse is too high and do not use strong narcotics for any type of arthritis pain. Others limit narcotic prescriptions to short periods, such as a few days—in which case a fentanyl patch, because it does not work quickly, would not usually be useful. Other physicians prescribe strong narcotics only when devastating arthritis problems are causing severe pain that cannot be controlled by other treatments. Most rheumatologists do not use strong narcotics for fibromyalgia or chronic lower back pain.

A clue to addictive behavior is if you are trying to get bigger doses of the drug and are not really using the bigger doses to control pain. The risk of addiction is higher in people who themselves, or whose family members, have had an addiction problem (alcohol or drugs). I have a few rules for my patients about narcotic prescriptions.

1. Use narcotics only for pain, not to feel good.
2. If you don't have pain, don't take them.
3. Get all your narcotic prescriptions from one doctor and from one pharmacy.
4. Escalating the dose can be an early sign of a problem.
5. Never sell, swap, or hoard narcotics.
6. If you are in the position of wanting to fool doctors or do illegal things such as forging signatures to get narcotic prescriptions, things are way out of control and you need to speak with your physician about getting help.

FLEXERIL (SEE CYCLOBENZAPRINE)

FLUOXETINE (*PROZAC*; SEE ***PROFILES OF COMMON ANTIDEPRESSANT DRUGS*** UNDER AMITRIPTYLINE)

FLURBIPROFEN

Brand Name

Ansaid.

Drug Family

Flurbiprofen is a nonsteroidal anti-inflammatory drug (NSAID). There are two big groups of NSAIDs, divided by whether they inhibit both cyclo-oxygenase (COX) enzymes, COX-1 and COX-2, or are more selective for COX-2. Flurbiprofen inhibits both COX-1 and COX-2.

Families of Arthritis Problems Prescribed For

NSAIDs are used to treat all kinds of pain and inflammation, whether they affect the joints or not. NSAIDs are used to treat many kinds of arthritis problems, such as RA, osteoarthritis, and bursitis. NSAIDs decrease pain and inflammation, but they do not change the progression of arthritis.

How It Works

Most NSAIDs inhibit the enzymes COX-1 and COX-2. Inhibiting these cyclo-oxygenase enzymes decreases the formation of chemicals called prostaglandins. Decreasing the prostaglandins made by COX-2 is anti-inflammatory, which is usually why we use NSAIDs. Inhibiting COX-1 makes platelets in your blood less sticky, which is why aspirin is used to prevent heart attacks. COX-1 also protects the stomach from ulcers, and blocking COX-1 may be why the risk of peptic ulcers is increased with many NSAIDs.

Avoid

Do not take flurbiprofen if you are allergic to it. People who have had a serious allergic reaction (swelling of the face and tongue, and wheezing) to one NSAID can have the same reaction with other NSAIDs. People with asthma or nasal polyps are more likely to be allergic to NSAIDs. NSAIDs are avoided if someone has an active peptic ulcer, is bleeding, or is pregnant.

Take Precautions

- NSAIDs can cause fluid retention and can worsen heart failure and high blood pressure.
- Some people have a higher risk for peptic ulcers caused by NSAIDs. Risk factors are being older than 65 years, having had a previous peptic ulcer, having had a previous bleeding ulcer, and taking a corticosteroid. In people at higher risk for peptic ulcers caused by NSAIDs, most rheumatologists would avoid an NSAID, if possible. If this is not possible, then prescribing misoprostol (see MISOPROSTOL—*Cytotec*) or a proton pump inhibitor (see OMEPRAZOLE—*Prilosec*) to protect against peptic ulcers caused by NSAIDs is an option. Another option is to use a COX-2 selective NSAID (see CELECOXIB—*Celebrex* and ROFECOXIB—*Vioxx*). None of these choices is foolproof, and peptic ulcers can still happen.
- NSAIDs have to be used carefully in people who have asthma, a bleeding problem, or liver or kidney problems.
- If you are taking NSAIDs regularly, blood tests will be done from time to time to check your blood count (in case you are losing blood slowly from an ulcer that you may not know about), your creatinine (for kidney function), and liver enzymes. People taking diuretics ("water pills") or ACE (angiotensin converting enzyme) inhibitors—a family of drugs that lowers blood pressure—and people with diabetes, heart failure, or existing kidney problems are more likely to have kidney problems caused by NSAIDs. These people may need more frequent blood tests to check their kidney function.

Side Effects

See NSAIDs.

Interactions with Other Drugs

See NSAIDs.

Important Information

- Taking NSAIDs with food is a good idea and may protect you from indigestion, but it does not prevent peptic ulcers.
- To minimize your GI risks, use the lowest effective dose of an NSAID.
- One of the signs that you may be bleeding from the stomach is if you have pitch-black bowel movements. Bowel movements with altered blood, in addition to being black, are also often runny and very smelly. If this happens, contact your doctor immediately.

Common Dose Sizes

Tablet: 50 mg, 100 mg.

Usual Adult Doses

The usual adult dose of flurbiprofen is 200 to 300 mg a day, divided into two or three doses.

Comments

See NSAIDs.

FOLIC ACID

Brand Name

Folvite.

Sometimes Called

Folate.

Drug Family

Folic acid is a vitamin.

Families of Arthritis Problems Prescribed For

Folic acid is used to protect against some of the side effects of methotrexate such as mouth ulcers, nausea, and changes in your blood count. It may also decrease the risk of liver problems with methotrexate.

How It Works

Folic acid blocks the effects of methotrexate in some cells and helps prevent side effects. In the doses used, folic acid does not block the effect of methotrexate on RA.

Avoid

Do not take folic acid if you have a vitamin B_{12} deficiency that has not been corrected.

Take Precautions

- If your doctor thinks you may be deficient in vitamin B_{12} a blood test can be done to check this before you start folic acid. In most people this is not required.

Side Effects

There are very few side effects from folic acid.

Rare: A rash and feeling flushed are rare. In people who are deficient in vitamin B_{12}, folic acid can speed up nerve damage caused by vitamin B_{12} deficiency. This is very rare.

Important Information

- Do not mix up your folic acid pills and your methotrexate pills. Methotrexate is usually taken once a week, and folic acid is usually taken every day.

Common Dose Sizes

Tablet: 0.1 mg, 0.4 mg, 0.8 mg, 1 mg.

Usual Adult Doses

Most rheumatologists use folic acid in doses of 1 mg a day to protect against the side effects of methotrexate. If someone is still having side effects caused by methotrexate, a higher dose can be tried. Some rheumatologists give one big dose of folic acid—say, 7 mg—on one day of the week. I prefer the daily dose.

Comments

Most people who take methotrexate for an arthritis problem also get folic acid, even if they have no side effects from the methotrexate. Some recent information shows that high homocysteine levels in the blood are a risk factor for coronary heart disease. Folic acid lowers homocysteine levels, and although there is no proof yet that folic acid prevents coronary heart disease, this is another potential benefit of folic acid treatment.

FOLINIC ACID

Brand Name

Wellcovorin.

Sometimes Called

Leucovorin, Tetrahydrofolate.

Drug Family

Folinic acid is a vitamin.

Families of Arthritis Problems Prescribed For

Folinic acid is sometimes used to protect against some of the side effects of methotrexate, such as mouth ulcers, nausea, and changes in your blood count. It may also decrease the risk of liver problems with methotrexate. Most rheumatologists prefer to use folic acid to prevent methotrexate side effects. Folinic acid is used to treat methotrexate toxicity. It is sometimes given as an injection to someone who has high levels of methotrexate in their blood and who has serious side effects from methotrexate, such as a drop in the white blood cell count. In some countries there are experimental protocols in which very high doses of methotrexate are given by injection and then, after a few days, the effects of methotrexate are reversed by giving folinic acid.

How It Works

High doses of methotrexate block the formation of folinic acid. Folinic acid tablets or injection replaces your folinic acid and block the effects of methotrexate.

Avoid

Do not take folinic acid if you have a vitamin B_{12} deficiency that has not been corrected.

Side Effects

There are very few side effects from folinic acid.

Rare: A rash and feeling flushed are rare. In people who are deficient in vitamin B_{12}, folinic acid can speed up nerve damage caused by vitamin B_{12} deficiency.

Usual Adult Doses

After high doses of methotrexate, overdose of methotrexate, or if the blood levels of methotrexate are high because of poor kidney function, folinic acid will be given as an injection in a dose that depends on how severe the problem is.

Different doses of folinic acid tablets have been used to prevent methotrexate side effects. One of the most common methods is to give equal doses of folinic acid and methotrexate once a week, but to delay the folinic acid, taking it four hours after the methotrexate.

Comments

Folinic acid has been used to prevent side effects caused by methotrexate but has largely been replaced by folic acid because there is more information showing that folic acid works. Folic acid is also cheaper, and there is a concern that folinic acid is more likely than folic acid to block some of the anti-inflammatory effects of methotrexate.

FOSAMAX (SEE ALENDRONATE)

GABAPENTIN

Brand Name

Neurontin.

Drug Family

Gabapentin belongs to the family of antiseizure medicines.

Families of Arthritis Problems Prescribed For

Gabapentin is approved by the FDA for the treatment of epilepsy, but it is also used to treat a wide range of pain problems, particularly pain caused by nerve damage.

How It Works

We do not know how gabapentin works to relieve some types of pain.

Avoid

Do not take gabapentin if you are allergic to it.

Side Effects

Gabapentin causes few side effects.

Uncommon: Sleepiness, dizziness, double vision, poor balance, fatigue, and GI side effects.

Rare: A low white blood cell count.

Interactions with Other Drugs

Gabapentin has few interactions with other drugs.

Cimetidine *(Tagamet):* The blood levels of gabapentin can be increased by cimetidine.

Important Information

- Don't take more than the prescribed dose of gabapentin.
- Don't drink alcohol while you are taking gabapentin.
- Gabapentin may cause drowsiness and affect your concentration when driving and performing other tasks.

Common Dose Sizes

Tablet: 100 mg, 300 mg, 400 mg.

Usual Adult Doses

The usual starting adult dose of gabapentin is one 300 mg tablet taken at night. The effective dose for pain control varies between 300 mg and 1,800 mg a day, usually divided into three doses.

Comments

Gabapentin is not used to control pain caused by arthritis. More often it is used to treat chronic pain that seems to have no specific cause or pain caused by nerve damage, as can happen in some people with what is called a "peripheral neuropathy" (often related to diabetes).

GAMMA GLOBULIN

Brand Name

Gamimune, Gammagard, Iveegam, Polygam, Sandoglobulin.

Sometimes Called

Intravenous immune globulin (IVIG).

Drug Family

Gamma globulin is an immunoglobulin, one of the proteins in blood that fights infection.

Families of Arthritis Problems Prescribed For

Gamma globulin is often given to people who, usually because of an inherited problem, do not make enough of their own gamma globulins. Gamma globulin is also used to treat idiopathic thrombocytopenic purpura, or ITP (an autoimmune problem in which the platelet count is very low because the platelets are destroyed by antibodies against them), Kawasaki disease (a rare problem with fever, rash, and swollen lymph glands, usually occurring in children), and some rare types of nerve damage such as Guillain Barré syndrome and chronic inflammatory demyelinating polyneuropathy. Gamma globulin has also sometimes been used to treat some autoimmune problems that are not responding to other treatment, but the evidence supporting this type of treatment is limited. It is occasionally used in people with vasculitis, rheumatoid arthritis, dermatomyositis, and systemic lupus erythematosus.

How It Works

In people with inherited deficiencies of gamma globulin and who have low levels of immunoglobulin, the replacement gamma globulin restores their levels. In autoimmune problems we are not sure how gamma globulin works.

Avoid

Do not receive gamma globulin if you are allergic to it. People who have an inherited low level of one of the immunoglobulins, called IgA, are more likely to have allergies to gamma globulin unless they are treated with preparations of gamma globulin that have little or no IgA.

Side Effects

Common: Feeling flushed, a rapid heartbeat, chills, and a feeling of shortness of breath can be felt during the infusion. These usually settle if the speed of the infusion is slowed down.

Less common: Low blood pressure, a serious allergic reaction, and aseptic meningitis (inflammation of the lining of the brain) are less common.

Rare: Gamma globulin is made from pooled human blood products, so there is a potential risk of transmitting a virus infection. Careful precautions are taken to make sure that IVIG does not carry any viral infections. Outbreaks, particularly of hepatitis C, have occurred with preparations that were not adequately sterilized, but these are rare.

Usual Adult Doses

For most autoimmune problems, 500 mg to 1 g per kg body weight is given intravenously slowly over a few hours.

Comments

Gamma globulin is prepared from pooled human plasma, and although the risk of getting an infection from viruses that we know about is very small, it is still a theoretical worry that there may be viruses we don't know about. Gamma globulin is expensive. There are few good studies in people with arthritis-related problems, such as dermatomyositis and vasculitis, to help us decide if IVIG is effective and which types of problems it may help. For all of these reasons, gamma globulin is only occasionally used to treat arthritis-related problems, usually when they are not responding to other treatments.

GLUCOSAMINE AND CHONDROITIN SULFATE

You can buy glucosamine and chondroitin sulfate as dietary supplements that are labeled "This product is not intended to diagnose, treat, cure, or prevent any disease." Most people who buy glucosamine or chondroitin use them to treat a medical problem—arthritis. Products such as these that fall somewhere between what we think of as medicines and what we think of as dietary supplements are sometimes called nutraceuticals.

Drug Family

Glucosamine and chondroitin sulfate are substances found in your joints, which, with other raw materials, are the building blocks of cartilage. Cartilage is the shock absorber in your joints that also helps the joints glide smoothly.

Families of Arthritis Problems Prescribed For

Most people who take glucosamine or chondroitin sulfate take it on their own, often without their doctor knowing about it, to treat all types of arthritis. The clinical trials that suggest that glucosamine is effective have studied people with osteoarthritis.

How It Works

We are not sure how these products work. It may not be a simple case of them replacing the raw materials that make up cartilage. They may also have anti-inflammatory effects.

Comments

There has been a lot of hype about glucosamine and some overenthusiastic claims. The evidence shows that glucosamine improves the symptoms of osteoarthritis (OA), sometimes as much as a low dose of an NSAID. There are more studies done with glucosamine sulphate than with glucosamine hydrochloride. It is fashionable to combine glucosamine and chondroitin sulfate, and there are several products with this combination. The combination of glucosamine and chondroitin sulfate has not been well studied, and it is not clear how much extra benefit chondroitin adds to glucosamine.

I am enthusiastic about any new treatment for OA that may be as effective as acetaminophen or an NSAID, particularly if the new treatment is safer.

My concerns are:

1. Many of the clinical studies have been small and lasted only a few weeks. In some of these studies, the drugs seemed to be effective, but not all the studies were very well designed. Glucosamine and chondroitin seem to be very safe, but we don't know much about their long-term safety.
2. There are worries about the quality control of some nutraceuticals. In the past products have not always contained the amount of drug that the label said they did.

From the limited information available, my thinking is that glucosamine, in a dose of 500 mg three times a day, is probably effective for reducing the pain from OA in some people, and it is probably safe. There is preliminary information from one study that glucosamine may slow down cartilage loss. If it does, this could be very important.

It is unfortunate that there are treatments that may be helpful for arthritis problems, but we do not know how effective or how safe they are. Until careful clinical trials are done, we won't know the answers to these questions.

GOLD INJECTIONS

There are two types of gold injection available, Aurothioglucose and Gold Sodium Thiomalate.

Brand Names

Solganal—Aurothioglucose; *Myochrysine* (discontinued), *Aurolate*—Gold Sodium Thiomalate.

Sometimes Called

Injectable gold.

Drug Family

Gold is a disease-modifying antirheumatic drug (DMARD).

Families of Arthritis Problems Prescribed For

Gold injections are most often used as a DMARD to treat rheumatoid arthritis. They are also sometimes used for psoriatic arthritis.

How It Works

We are not sure how gold works in rheumatoid arthritis. Gold affects some of your white blood cell functions, but it does not suppress your immune system and so does not increase your risk of infection.

Avoid

Avoid gold if you are allergic to it, if you have had serious bone-marrow problems, or if your kidney function is poor. Gold is avoided in pregnancy.

Take Precautions

• Gold can cause, and worsen, skin problems such as dermatitis or eczema. If you develop a skin rash, stop the drug and contact your doctor.

• Gold must be used cautiously in people with decreased liver or kidney function.

• Your blood count and urine will be tested regularly. These tests are usually done fairly frequently, often every week, after you start gold injections. After a while they will be done once a month. The white cell count and platelet count in your blood will be checked, and if they drop significantly, gold may need to be stopped. Your urine will be checked for protein and, if you start to show protein in the urine, gold may need to be stopped.

• Avoid spending time in the sun, because gold can increase your skin's sensitivity to sunlight.

Side Effects

Side effects are common with gold injections, and many people who start gold injections have to stop within a couple of years because they get side effects.

Common: Itching, a skin rash, mouth ulcers, a metallic taste, and protein in the urine are fairly common.

Rare: Much less common, but more serious, are a severe skin rash with skin peeling, other serious allergic reactions, serious bone marrow problems with a low white cell count or low platelet count, liver problems, peripheral nerve problems, and fever and lung problems. There is a side effect called a "nitritoid reaction" that happens in some people immediately after a gold injection—they flush and feel faint. This is not an allergic reaction, but some people cannot take gold shots because of it. Nitritoid reactions are more common with the gold sodium thiomalate preparation.

Interactions with Other Drugs

Other DMARDs: Penicillamine and gold are not combined.

Important Information

- Monitoring is important. Don't skip your lab checkups.
- Gold works slowly, but if you have had no response after six months of treatment, it is time to think about and another DMARD.
- If you develop a skin rash, stop the gold and contact your doctor.

Common Dose Sizes

Aurothioglucose injection: 50 mg/ml (10 ml vial).
Gold sodium thiomalate injection: 50 mg/ml (10 ml vial).

Usual Adult Doses

The usual adult starting dose for gold injections is a 10 mg intramuscular (IM) dose the first week. This low dose is given to make sure you are not allergic to gold. The next week a 25 mg IM dose is given, and after that the dose is 50 mg a week IM until the RA responds or until a total dose of 1 g has been given (about twenty weeks). If your arthritis has not responded, your doctor might recommend another DMARD. If your RA responds to gold, the injections can be given less often—usually every two weeks for a couple of months and then, if things are going well, every three or four weeks.

Comments

In the 1980s many people with RA were on gold injections, and many rheumatologists had special "gold clinics." Now gold has mostly been replaced by safer and more effective treatments, and most rheumatologists have only a handful of patients who are still getting gold injections. There are a few people who respond very well to gold and who do not develop side effects. But in many people gold is only partly effective and side effects are common.

Gold works slowly, and it may be six to twelve weeks before you notice an improvement in your arthritis. If your arthritis has not responded after three or four months of gold treatment, your doctor might recommend another DMARD. As far as the choice between oral gold and gold injection goes, I think that oral gold is probably less effective than gold injections, but oral gold also causes serious side effects less often.

GOLD, ORAL (SEE AURANOFIN) (*Ridaura*)

HYALURONAN INJECTIONS

Two types of hyaluronan injections are available: SODIUM HYALURONATE *(Hyalgan)* and HYLAN GF 20 *(Synvisc)*.

Brand Names

Hyalgan: SODIUM HYALURONATE, *Synvisc:* HYLAN GF 20

Sometimes Called

Viscosupplements, Hyaluronic acid.

Drug Family

This is a unique family of medicines that may improve the lubrication of joints.

Families of Arthritis Problems Prescribed For

Hyaluronan injections are used to treat osteoarthritis of the knee.

How It Works

No one is exactly sure how they work. Hyaluronic acid is found in normal joint fluid and improves the viscosity of the fluid so that it cushions the joints better. The initial idea was that when they were injected into the joint these drugs replaced the lubricant, hyaluronic acid, in joint fluid. We now know that the explanation is not as simple as this. The hyaluronan that is injected does not stay in the joint very long because it is quickly taken up by the body. This means that hyaluronan injections are not working simply as lubricants but have other effects, probably anti-inflammatory effects.

Avoid

Do not get SODIUM HYALURONATE or HYLAN GF 20 injections if you are allergic to them. Joint injections are not given if you have a skin infection close to the joint.

Take Precautions

- These drugs have been tested for osteoarthritis of the knee. There is little information about using them in other joints.
- Caution is recommended in people who are allergic to eggs, feathers, or bird proteins because they may be allergic to the injections.

Side Effects

Common: Knee pain and swelling or warmth and redness of the skin at the injection site can occur. Usually this is not a problem, but sometimes the knee joint can flare and become very hot, swollen, and painful.

Rare: There is a very small risk of an infection getting into any joint when it is injected. This risk is from the injection itself and not from the drugs injected. Allergic reactions to hyaluronan injections can occur.

Interactions with Other Drugs

The manufacturers recommend that other drugs should not be injected into the knee at the same time as the hyaluronan.

Important Information

- If your knee becomes red, hot, and swollen and you have difficulty moving it after you have had an intra-articular injection, you should call your doctor. This can happen as a reaction to the injection but can also be a sign of an infection in the knee.
- To get the most benefit, you need to complete the course of injections.
- After the injection, rest your knee for a day or two by avoiding strenuous activities.

Common Dose Sizes

These injections come in prepacked syringes for your physician to inject into your knee joint.

Usual Adult Doses

SODIUM HYALURONATE *(Hyalgan):* The usual dose is five injections into the knee joint, one week apart.

HYLAN GF 20 *(Synvisc):* The usual dose is three injections into the knee joint, one week apart.

Comments

Hyaluronan injections can help some people for months after the course of injections, but on average the responses to treatment are unimpressive. The treatment can help symptoms—pain and stiffness—but does not affect the underlying arthritis problem. The injections may be about as effective as an NSAID, but the effects wear off over time. Many patients are not comfortable with having several injections into their knee, and the course of treatment is expensive, particularly when you add the cost of the drugs and the cost of getting the injections. Hyaluronan injections are sometimes used to try to help someone with osteoarthritis (OA) of the knee who is not responding to an NSAID and who is not yet ready for knee-replacement surgery. If you have OA of the knee, don't forget about all the other things that can help, such as losing weight if you are overweight, an exercise program to strengthen your quadriceps, and using heat or cold to relieve pain and stiffness.

HYALURONATE (*HYALGAN*) (SEE HYALURONAN INJECTIONS)

HYALGAN (HYALURONATE) (SEE HYALURONAN INJECTIONS)

HYDROCODONE (SEE ACETAMINOPHEN + NARCOTICS)

HYDROCORTISONE (SEE CORTICOSTEROIDS)

HYDROXYCHLOROQUINE AND CHLOROQUINE PHOSPHATE

Hydroxychloroquine *(Plaquenil)* and chloroquine *(Aralen)* are very similar. Hydroxychloroquine causes fewer side effects and is used more often than chloroquine.

Brand Names

Plaquenil—hydroxychloroquine, *Aralen*—chloroquine.

Sometimes Called

Antimalarials.

Drug Family

These drugs are disease-modifying antirheumatic drugs (DMARDs) and are also used to treat and prevent certain types of malaria infection (antimalarials).

Families of Arthritis Problems Prescribed For

Antimalarials are used as DMARDs in RA and to treat the skin and joint problems in people with systemic lupus erythematosus (SLE). They are occasionally used for psoriatic arthritis.

How It Works

We do not know how antimalarials work in autoimmune problems. They alter the immune system but do not suppress it, so there is no increased risk of infections.

Avoid

Do not take hydroxychloroquine or chloroquine if you are allergic to them. If possible, antimalarials are avoided in pregnancy. There is some evidence that antimalarials can damage the developing baby, but there are also reports of people with lupus having taken hydroxychloroquine throughout pregnancy without problems. The risk to the developing baby from a lupus flare-up, which may be caused by stopping hydroxychloroquine, may be greater than the risk from the medicine. If you are planning a pregnancy and are taking hydroxychloroquine, this is something that you will have to discuss with your rheumatologist and obstetrician.

Take Precautions

- Caution is needed when people who have liver problems, psoriasis, or a rare problem called porphyria take antimalarials. Antimalarials, although they are sometimes used to treat the arthritis that can go with psoriasis, can sometimes make the psoriasis skin rash worse.
- Eye testing is advised every six to twelve months.

Side Effects

Hydroxychloroquine is one of the best-tolerated DMARDs. Serious side effects are very rare.

Common: Headache, blurred vision, and mild GI symptoms such as indigestion, gas, or nausea can occur. The blurred vision tends to be worse when people start hydroxychloroquine and is not caused by eye damage. What happens is that the muscles in the eye that change the size of the pupil become a little sluggish. This effect usually wears off.

Rare: Skin rashes, often with darkening of the skin, can occur. Hydroxychloroquine and chloroquine cause two eye problems. The first is small flecks in the clear layer over the lens of the eye, called the cornea. The second, toxicity to the nerve cell layer at the back of the eye (the retina), is rare but can cause irreversible loss of vision. The retinal toxicity, on the rare occasions that it has occurred, has not usually happened suddenly but has come on gradually after someone has been on hydroxychloroquine or chloroquine for a long time, usually many years. This is why you will be asked to have your eyes checked once or twice a year. If the problem is spotted early and hydroxychloroquine is stopped, the problem does not usually progress. The risk of retinal problems is higher in people who are older than 70 years, people with poor liver or kidney function, and people who take a dose of hydroxychloroquine higher than 6 mg per kg a day. Retinal toxicity is very rare, and most rheumatologists can remember only a couple of people who they thought had this problem.

Hydroxychloroquine and chloroquine can also damage muscles. This can cause weakness, and heart failure if the heart muscles are affected. If you are taking antimalarials and start having serious heart or muscle problems, it is worth reminding your physicians that antimalarials can cause muscle problems. This is a very uncommon problem. Again, most rheumatologists can recall only a handful of people in whom this may have been a problem.

Other rare side effects are blood problems, ear problems causing dizziness or deafness, and nerve damage.

Interactions with Other Drugs

Penicillamine: When hydroxychloroquine is combined with penicillamine, also a DMARD, side effects can be more frequent.

Important Information

- Serious eye problems from hydroxychloroquine virtually never happen in people who have taken a dose of less than 6 mg/kg/day. This dose is based on lean body weight or ideal body weight, not your actual weight. So if you are a 5-foot-10-inch-tall person and weigh 220 lbs (100 kg), your ideal body weight would be around 160 lbs (about 70 kg) and your dose of hydroxychloroquine would be 400 mg a day, not 600 mg a day.
- It is controversial how often people need eye checks while they are taking hydroxychloroquine. The eye problem

is so rare, particularly with a dose of hydroxychloroquine less than 6 mg/kg/day, that some experts think that eye checks once or twice a year are unnecessary. The strictest guidelines recommend eye checks every six months, but in practice many people at low risk are checked less often.

Common Dose Sizes

Tablets: Hydroxychloroquine 200 mg.
Tablets: Chloroquine 250 mg.

Usual Adult Doses

Hydroxychloroquine: The usual adult dose of hydroxychloroquine is 5 mg to 6 mg per kg lean body weight. The dose is usually 200 mg or 400 mg a day.

Chloroquine: The usual adult dose of chloroquine is up to 4 mg per kg lean body weight. The dose is usually 250 mg a day.

Comments

Hydroxychloroquine and chloroquine are very similar. Hydroxychloroquine may be slightly less effective than chloroquine, but it causes side effects less often and is used for arthritis problems much more often than chloroquine is.

In RA, hydroxychloroquine is a relatively weak DMARD and is useful for people with very mild or early problems. In people with more severe RA, hydroxychloroquine is used in combination with other DMARDs, such as methotrexate or sulfasalazine. In people with SLE, hydroxychloroquine is useful for the skin and joint problems that lupus can cause. I try to get almost all my patients with SLE taking hydroxychloroquine because I think it stabilizes other lupus problems as well. There is some evidence that hydroxychloroquine may lower cholesterol by a small amount.

HYLAN GF 20 (SYNVISC) *(SEE HYALURONAN INJECTIONS)*

IBUPROFEN

Brand Names

Advil, Genpril, Ibuprin, Motrin, and *Nuprin.*

Drug Family

Ibuprofen is a nonsteroidal anti-inflammatory drug (NSAID). There are two big groups of NSAIDs, divided by whether they inhibit both cyclo-oxygenase (COX) enzymes, COX-1 and COX-2, or are more selective for COX-2. Ibuprofen inhibits both COX-1 and COX-2.

Families of Arthritis Problems Prescribed For

NSAIDs are used to treat all kinds of pain and inflammation, whether they affect the joints or not. NSAIDs are used to treat many kinds of arthritis problems, such as RA, gout, ankylosing spondylitis, osteoarthritis, and bursitis. NSAIDs decrease pain and inflammation, but they do not change the progression of arthritis.

How It Works

Most NSAIDs inhibit the enzymes COX-1 and COX-2. Inhibiting these cyclo-oxygenase enzymes decreases the formation of chemicals called prostaglandins. Decreasing the prostaglandins made by COX-2 is anti-inflammatory, which is usually why we use NSAIDs. Inhibiting COX-1 makes platelets in your blood less sticky, which is why aspirin is used to treat heart attacks. COX-1 also protects the stomach from ulcers, and blocking COX-1 may be why the risk of peptic ulcers is increased with many NSAIDs.

Avoid

Do not take ibuprofen if you are allergic to it. People who have had a serious allergic reaction (swelling of the face and tongue, and wheezing) to one NSAID can have the same reaction to other NSAIDs. People with asthma or nasal polyps are more likely to be allergic to NSAIDs. NSAIDs are avoided if someone has an active peptic ulcer, is bleeding, or is pregnant.

Take Precautions

- NSAIDs can cause fluid retention and can worsen heart failure and high blood pressure.
- Some people are at higher risk for peptic ulcers caused by NSAIDs. Risk factors are being older than 65 years, having had a previous peptic ulcer, having had a previous bleeding ulcer, and taking a corticosteroid. In people at higher risk for peptic ulcers caused by NSAIDs, most rheumatologists would avoid an NSAID, if possible. If this is not possible, then prescribing misoprostol (see MISOPROSTOL—*Cytotec*) or a proton pump inhibitor (see OMEPRAZOLE—*Prilosec*) to protect against peptic ulcers caused by NSAIDs is an option. Another option is to use a COX-2 selective NSAID (see CELECOXIB—*Celebrex* and ROFECOXIB—*Vioxx*). None of these choices is foolproof, and peptic ulcers can still happen.
- NSAIDs have to be used carefully in people who have asthma, a bleeding problem, or liver or kidney problems.
- If you are taking NSAIDs regularly, blood tests will be done from time to time to check your blood count (in case you are losing blood slowly from an ulcer that you may not know about), your creatinine (for kidney function), and liver

enzymes. People taking diuretics ("water pills") or ACE (angiotensin converting enzyme) inhibitors—a family of drugs that lowers blood pressure—and people with diabetes, heart failure, or existing kidney problems are more likely to have kidney problems caused by NSAIDs. These people may need more frequent blood tests to check their kidney function.

Side Effects

See NSAIDs.

Interactions with Other Drugs

See NSAIDs.

Important Information

- Taking NSAIDs with food is a good idea and may protect you from indigestion, but it does not prevent peptic ulcers.
- To minimize your GI risks, use the lowest effective dose of an NSAID.
- One of the signs that you may be bleeding from the stomach is if you have pitch-black bowel movements. Bowel movements with altered blood, in addition to being black, are also often runny and very smelly. If this happens, contact your doctor immediately.

Common Dose Sizes

Tablet: 200 mg, 300 mg, 400 mg, 600 mg, 800 mg.

Usual Adult Doses

The usual adult dose of ibuprofen is 400 mg to 800 mg three to four times a day. The usual maximum dose is 3.2 g a day.

Comments

See NSAIDs.

Ibuprofen may have less GI toxicity than other nonselective NSAIDs, but this may be because lower doses of ibuprofen have been included in studies that have looked at this.

IMIPRAMINE (*TOFRANIL;* SEE ***PROFILES OF COMMON ANTIDEPRESSANT DRUGS*** UNDER AMITRIPTYLINE)

IMURAN (SEE AZATHIOPRINE)

INDOCIN (SEE INDOMETHACIN)

INDOMETHACIN

Brand Name

Indocin.

Drug Family

Indomethacin is a nonsteroidal anti-inflammatory drug (NSAID). There are two big groups of NSAIDs, divided by whether they inhibit both cyclo-oxygenase (COX) enzymes, COX-1 and COX-2, or are more selective for COX-2. Indomethacin inhibits both COX-1 and COX-2.

Families of Arthritis Problems Prescribed For

NSAIDs are used to treat all kinds of pain and inflammation, whether they affect the joints or not. NSAIDs are used to treat many kinds of arthritis problems, such as RA, gout, ankylosing spondylitis, reactive arthritis, osteoarthritis, and bursitis. NSAIDs decrease pain and inflammation, but they do not change the progression of arthritis.

How It Works

Most NSAIDs inhibit the enzymes COX-1 and COX-2. Inhibiting these cyclo-oxygenase enzymes decreases the formation of chemicals called prostaglandins. Decreasing the prostaglandins made by COX-2 is anti-inflammatory, which is usually why we use NSAIDs. Inhibiting COX-1 makes platelets in your blood less sticky, which is why aspirin is used to treat heart attacks. COX-1 also protects the stomach from ulcers, and blocking COX-1 may be why the risk of peptic ulcers is increased with many NSAIDs.

Avoid

Do not take indomethacin if you are allergic to it. People who have had a serious allergic reaction (swelling of the face and tongue, and wheezing) to one NSAID can have the same reaction with other NSAIDs. People with asthma or nasal polyps are more likely to be allergic to NSAIDs. NSAIDs are avoided if someone has an active peptic ulcer, is bleeding, or is pregnant.

Take Precautions

- NSAIDs can cause fluid retention and can worsen heart failure and high blood pressure.
- Some people are at higher risk for peptic ulcers caused by NSAIDs. Risk factors are being older than 65 years, having had a previous peptic ulcer, having had a previous bleeding ulcer, and taking a corticosteroid. In people at higher risk for peptic ulcers caused by NSAIDs, most rheumatologists would avoid an NSAID, if possible. If this is not possible, prescribing misoprostol (see MISOPROSTOL—*Cytotec*) or a proton pump inhibitor (see OMEPRAZOLE—*Prilosec*) to protect against peptic ulcers caused by NSAIDs is an option. Another option is to use a COX-2 selective NSAID (see CELECOXIB—

Celebrex and ROFECOXIB—*Vioxx*). None of these choices is foolproof, and peptic ulcers can still happen.

• NSAIDs have to be used carefully in people who have asthma, a bleeding problem, or liver or kidney problems.

• If you are taking NSAIDs regularly, blood tests will be done from time to time to check your blood count (in case you are losing blood slowly from an ulcer that you may not know about), your creatinine (for kidney function), and liver enzymes. People taking diuretics ("water pills") or ACE (angiotensin converting enzyme) inhibitors—a family of drugs that lowers blood pressure—and people with diabetes, heart failure, or existing kidney problems are more likely to have kidney problems caused by NSAIDs. These people may need more frequent blood tests to check their kidney function.

Side Effects

See NSAIDs.

Indomethacin seems to cause headaches and a "spacy" feeling more frequently than some of the other NSAIDs.

Interactions with Other Drugs

See NSAIDs.

Important Information

• Taking NSAIDs with food is a good idea and may protect you from indigestion, but it does not prevent peptic ulcers.

• To minimize your GI risks, use the lowest effective dose of an NSAID.

• One of the signs that you may be bleeding from the stomach is if you have pitch-black bowel movements. Bowel movements with altered blood, in addition to being black, are also often runny and very smelly. If this happens, contact your doctor immediately.

Common Dose Sizes
Capsule: 25 mg, 50 mg
Capsule, sustained-release: 75 mg.

Usual Adult Doses
The usual adult dose of indomethacin is 25 mg to 50 mg taken two to three times a day to a maximum of 150 mg a day. Sustained-release indomethacin (75 mg) is taken once or twice a day.

Comments
See NSAIDs.

Indomethacin may be slightly more effective than other NSAIDs for ankylosing spondylitis, Reiter's syndrome, and acute gout. But for most other problems, because side effects are more frequent with indomethacin, particularly in older people, other NSAIDs are usually tried first.

INFLIXIMAB

Brand Name
Remicade.

Sometimes Called
Tumor necrosis factor (TNF) antagonist.

Drug Family
Infliximab acts as a disease-modifying antirheumatic drug (DMARD) in RA.

Families of Arthritis Problems Prescribed For
Infliximab is used to treat rheumatoid arthritis and juvenile rheumatoid arthritis (JRA). Infliximab is used to treat RA in

people who are already taking methotrexate but whose RA has not responded completely. There are a few reports of TNF antagonists being used to treat vasculitis, but the information is very preliminary. Infliximab is approved for the treatment of Crohn's disease, a problem that causes inflammation of the bowel.

How It Works

Infliximab is a biological drug. It is an antibody designed to neutralize the effects of the cytokine TNF (tumor necrosis factor) that your body makes. Infliximab is an antibody against human TNF, but it was first made from a mouse antibody. The mouse antibody was then changed through genetic synthesis methods so that most of it has the structure of a human antibody. This was done so that your body, which recognizes human antibodies, does not develop antibodies against infliximab that could destroy it or cause allergic reactions. A few people do develop antibodies to infliximab. This happens less often in people who are also taking another drug that suppresses their immune system, such as methotrexate.

Avoid

Do not take infliximab if you are allergic to it or have an active infection. Infliximab is usually avoided in people who have had cancer, particularly lymphoma.

Take Precautions

- Infliximab can suppress your immune response; take any infections seriously and have them treated early.
- If you develop a serious infection, stop infliximab and contact your doctor.
- Caution is advised in people with multiple sclerosis (MS) or optic neuritis.

Side Effects

Infliximab, so far, is remarkably safe.

Common: Infliximab is given as an intravenous infusion. Minor side effects during the infusion are fairly common. These include fever, chills, rash, and itching. These infusion reactions are seldom serious, and few people have to stop treatment because of them.

Less common: Infliximab is used with methotrexate to treat RA. The combination of infliximab and methotrexate can cause a mild elevation of the liver enzyme tests more often than methotrexate alone does.

Rare: A serious allergic reaction to infliximab is rare but can happen. Infections, some serious, have occurred in people taking infliximab, but it is not clear if infliximab increases the risks of infection, and if it does, by how much. There is no evidence that infliximab increases the risk of cancer, but cancer can take a long time to develop, so it will be several years before we have enough information about this. Some people, about 5 to 10 percent of those taking infliximab, will develop a positive antinuclear antibody (ANA) test. The ANA is a blood test that is positive in most people with lupus but is also positive in many healthy people. There is the worry that infliximab may increase the risk of autoimmune problems, such as lupus. So far very few people have developed a lupus-like problem. Bone marrow suppression resulting in low blood cell counts and neurological problems similar to multiple sclerosis have occurred with anti-TNF drugs, but they are very rare.

Interactions with Other Drugs

Vaccines: Live virus vaccines are avoided in people taking infliximab.

Important Information

- Avoid becoming pregnant while you are taking infliximab.
- Avoid immunizations (except for influenza and pneumonia immunization) unless discussed with your physician.
- Contact your doctor if you develop any serious or prolonged infection or fever.

Common Dose Sizes

Infliximab comes as a vial that contains 100 mg.

Usual Adult Doses

The usual adult dose of infliximab is 3 mg per kg body weight given as a slow intravenous infusion over two hours or longer. The infusion is repeated two weeks and six weeks after the first dose; after that it is given every eight weeks. People who get infliximab for RA are usually already taking methotrexate.

Comments

Biological drugs are likely to become widely used to treat RA. The TNF antagonists are very effective and, so far, very safe. Infliximab is used in combination with methotrexate. This means that it is a good option for people who are taking methotrexate and still have active RA. In clinical trials, about 30 percent of people who were poorly controlled on methotrexate alone and got infliximab plus methotrexate had a 50 percent or greater response in their overall RA activity. Unlike other DMARDs, people respond very quickly to anti-TNF drugs and often feel better within a couple of weeks. But as with all DMARDs, not everyone responds to anti-TNF treatment. Infliximab is not a good option for people who cannot take methotrexate. There are a couple of drawbacks with the drug.

1. Infliximab is given by intravenous injection. Most people don't find this a problem, but some find it inconvenient to spend several hours at the infusion center every eight weeks. The injections are given into a vein. In some people it can be difficult to find a vein to inject.
2. Infliximab is very expensive, costing at least ten times more than most traditional DMARD treatments. On the other hand, poorly controlled RA can be very expensive if one thinks of things such as decreased income, a poor quality of life, and joint-replacement surgery.
3. We are accumulating long-term information about side effects. At the moment TNF blockers seem to be unusually safe drugs. But we will only know the answers to the really important questions, such as the risks of cancer, in a few years time.

Anti-TNF drugs are a huge advance in the treatment of RA, but they are not for everyone. If you have mild or moderate RA that is well controlled with standard DMARDs, there is no advantage to switching to an anti-TNF drug. On the other hand, if you have RA that remains active, in spite of standard DMARD treatment or combination DMARD treatment, and if your health insurance covers anti-TNF treatment or you can afford it, this treatment could be for you.

There are two anti-TNF drugs on the market, etanercept *(Enbrel)* and infliximab *(Remicade)*. They work in different ways and are given differently. Etanercept is given as an injection under the skin twice a week and infliximab as an intravenous infusion at zero, two, and six weeks and then every eight weeks. It is standard practice to combine infliximab with methotrexate, mainly to suppress antibodies that your body could make against the drug. This is not the case with etanercept, which can be used alone, without methotrexate.

INTRAVENOUS IMMUNOGLOBULIN (IVIG) (SEE GAMMA GLOBULIN)

KENALOG (SEE CORTICOSTEROIDS, INTRA-ARTICULAR)

KETOPROFEN

Brand Names
Orudis, Oruvail.

Drug Family
Ketoprofen is a nonsteroidal anti-inflammatory drug (NSAID). There are two big groups of NSAIDs, divided by whether they inhibit both cyclo-oxygenase (COX) enzymes, COX-1 and COX-2, or are more selective for COX-2. Ketoprofen inhibits both COX-1 and COX-2.

Families of Arthritis Problems Prescribed For
NSAIDs are used to treat all kinds of pain and inflammation, whether they affect the joints or not. NSAIDs are used to treat many kinds of arthritis problems, such as RA, gout, ankylosing spondylitis, osteoarthritis, and bursitis. NSAIDs decrease pain and inflammation, but they do not change the progression of arthritis.

How It Works
Most NSAIDs inhibit the enzymes COX-1 and COX-2. Inhibiting these cyclo-oxygenase enzymes decreases the formation of chemicals called prostaglandins. Decreasing the prostaglandins made by COX-2 is anti-inflammatory, which is usually why we use NSAIDs. Inhibiting COX-1 makes

platelets in your blood less sticky, which is why aspirin is used to treat heart attacks. COX-1 also protects the stomach from ulcers, and blocking COX-1 may be why the risk of peptic ulcers is increased with many NSAIDs.

Avoid

Do not take ketoprofen if you are allergic to it. People who have had a serious allergic reaction (swelling of the face and tongue, and wheezing) to one NSAID can have the same reaction with other NSAIDs. People with asthma or nasal polyps are more likely to be allergic to NSAIDs. NSAIDs are avoided if someone has an active peptic ulcer, is bleeding, or is pregnant.

Take Precautions

- NSAIDs can cause fluid retention and can worsen heart failure and high blood pressure.
- Some people are at higher risk for peptic ulcers caused by NSAIDs. Risk factors are being older than 65 years, having had a previous peptic ulcer, having had a previous bleeding ulcer, and taking a corticosteroid. In people at higher risk for peptic ulcers caused by NSAIDs, most rheumatologists would avoid an NSAID, if possible. If this is not possible, then prescribing misoprostol (see MISOPROSTOL—*Cytotec*) or a proton pump inhibitor (see OMEPRAZOLE—*Prilosec*) to protect against peptic ulcers caused by NSAIDs is an option. Another option is to use a COX-2 selective NSAID (see CELECOXIB—*Celebrex* and ROFECOXIB—*Vioxx*). None of these choices is foolproof, and peptic ulcers can still happen.
- NSAIDs have to be used carefully in people who have asthma, a bleeding problem, or liver or kidney problems.
- If you are taking NSAIDs regularly, blood tests will be done from time to time to check your blood count (in case you are losing blood slowly from an ulcer that you may not know

about), your creatinine (for kidney function), and liver enzymes. People taking diuretics ("water pills") or ACE (angiotensin converting enzyme) inhibitors—a family of drugs that lowers blood pressure—and people with diabetes, heart failure, or existing kidney problems are more likely to have kidney problems caused by NSAIDs. These people may need more frequent blood tests to check their kidney function.

Side Effects

See NSAIDs.

Interactions with Other Drugs

See NSAIDs.

Important Information

- Taking NSAIDs with food is a good idea and may protect you from indigestion, but it does not prevent peptic ulcers.
- To minimize your GI risks, use the lowest effective dose of an NSAID.
- One of the signs that you may be bleeding from the stomach is if you have pitch-black bowel movements. Bowel movements with altered blood, in addition to being black, are also often runny and very smelly. If this happens, contact your doctor immediately.

Common Dose Sizes

Capsule: 25 mg, 50 mg, 75 mg.
Capsule, extended-release: 100 mg, 200 mg.

Usual Adult Doses

The usual adult dose of ketoprofen is 50 mg to 75 mg taken three or four times a day up to a maximum dose of 300 mg a day. The dose of the extended-release ketoprofen preparation is 200 mg once daily.

Comments

See NSAIDs.

KETOROLAC

Brand Name

Toradol.

Drug Family

Ketorolac is a nonsteroidal anti-inflammatory drug (NSAID). There are two big groups of NSAIDs, divided by whether they inhibit both cyclo-oxygenase (COX) enzymes, COX-1 and COX-2, or are more selective for COX-2. Ketorolac inhibits both COX-1 and COX-2.

Families of Arthritis Problems Prescribed For

Ketorolac is an NSAID, but it is used differently from most other NSAIDs. Ketorolac is used only for short periods to treat acute pain, such as pain after an operation or pain caused by a kidney stone.

How It Works

Most NSAIDs inhibit the enzymes COX-1 and COX-2. Inhibiting these cyclo-oxygenase enzymes decreases the formation of chemicals called prostaglandins. Decreasing the prostaglandins made by COX-2 is anti-inflammatory, which is usually why we use NSAIDs. Inhibiting COX-1 makes platelets in your blood less sticky, which is why aspirin is used to treat heart attacks. COX-1 also protects the stomach from ulcers, and blocking COX-1 may be why the risk of peptic ulcers is increased with many NSAIDs.

Avoid

Do not take ketorolac if you are allergic to it. People who have had a serious allergic reaction (swelling of the face and tongue, and wheezing) to one NSAID can have the same reaction with other NSAIDs. People with asthma or nasal polyps are more likely to be allergic to NSAIDs. NSAIDs are avoided if someone has an active peptic ulcer, is bleeding, or is pregnant.

Take Precautions

• NSAIDs can cause fluid retention and can worsen heart failure and high blood pressure.

• Some people are at higher risk for peptic ulcers caused by NSAIDs. Risk factors are being older than 65 years, having had a previous peptic ulcer, having had a previous bleeding ulcer, and taking a corticosteroid. In people at higher risk for peptic ulcers caused by NSAIDs, most rheumatologists would avoid an NSAID, if possible. If this is not possible, then prescribing misoprostol (see MISOPROSTOL—*Cytotec*) or a proton pump inhibitor (see OMEPRAZOLE—*Prilosec*) to protect against peptic ulcers caused by NSAIDs is an option. Another option is to use a COX-2 selective NSAID (see CELECOXIB—*Celebrex* and ROFECOXIB—*Vioxx*). None of these choices is foolproof, and peptic ulcers can still happen.

• NSAIDs have to be used carefully in people who have asthma, a bleeding problem, or liver or kidney problems.

• Ketorolac should not be used for more than five days because after that the risk of side effects goes up.

• NSAIDs can cause a decrease in kidney function. This shows up as an increase in the concentration of creatinine in your blood. People taking diuretics ("water pills") or ACE (angiotensin converting enzyme) inhibitors—a family of drugs that lowers blood pressure—and people with diabetes, heart failure, or existing kidney problems are more likely to have kidney problems caused by NSAIDs. These people may need more frequent blood tests to check their kidney function.

Side Effects

See NSAIDs.

The risk of side effects from ketorolac increases if it is used for more than a few days.

Interactions with Other Drugs

See NSAIDs.

Important Information

- Taking NSAIDs with food is a good idea and may protect you from indigestion, but it does not prevent peptic ulcers.
- To minimize your GI risks, use the lowest effective dose of an NSAID.
- One of the signs that you may be bleeding from the stomach is if you have pitch-black bowel movements. Bowel movements with altered blood, in addition to being black, are also often runny and very smelly. If this happens, contact your doctor immediately.

Common Dose Sizes

Tablet: 10 mg.

Usual Adult Doses

The usual adult dose of ketorolac is a 10 mg tablet taken three to four times a day, up to a maximum of 40 mg a day. Ketorolac should not be taken for more than five days.

Comments

Most people take NSAIDs for arthritis pain. Ketorolac,

because it is used for only a few days, is not suitable for chronic arthritis pain. If someone is already taking an NSAID, he should avoid ketorolac.

LANSOPRAZOLE (*PREVACID;* SEE ***PROFILES OF COMMON PROTON PUMP INHIBITORS*** UNDER OMEPRAZOLE)

LEFLUNOMIDE

Brand Name

Arava.

Drug Family

Leflunomide started off as an antirejection drug that was being developed for people who have organ transplants. Leflunomide stays in your body for a long time and affects your immune response, so it was developed as a disease-modifying antirheumatic drug (DMARD) for RA.

Families of Arthritis Problems Prescribed For

Leflunomide was approved by the FDA in 1998 as a DMARD to treat rheumatoid arthritis. There is some preliminary evidence showing that leflunomide may be useful for psoriatic arthritis and also to hold vasculitis in remission.

How It Works

Leflunomide blocks an enzyme that is important for the formation of pyrimidines, one of the building blocks of DNA. Lymphocytes, a type of white blood cell, are particularly sensitive to leflunomide. Leflunomide blocks your immune response by blocking pyrimidine synthesis in lymphocytes.

Avoid

Do not take leflunomide if you are allergic to it. People who have liver problems should not take leflunomide. Leflunomide is avoided in pregnancy (see Precautions). Most rheumatologists would avoid using leflunomide in people infected with HIV, hepatitis B, or hepatitis C.

Take Precautions

- Caution is needed in people with decreased liver or kidney function.
- Blood tests will be done to check your liver function tests, usually every four to eight weeks.
- Because leflunomide can suppress your immune system, you should take seriously any infections that you may get and have them treated early.
- Leflunomide, in pregnant animals, can damage the developing offspring. Make sure that you are not pregnant before you start taking leflunomide. Use reliable contraception while you are taking leflunomide. If you are a woman who can bear children and you stop taking leflunomide, you should take a course of cholestyramine (*Questran*). Cholestyramine is a type of resin that binds onto leflunomide in your gut and helps your body gets rid of leflunomide more quickly. Without a course of cholestyramine, leflunomide will stay in your body for two years or longer.

There is no information whether leflunomide affects the development of a baby conceived while a man is taking leflunomide. To be on the safe side, men who are taking leflunomide and want to start a family should stop leflunomide and take a course of cholestyramine.

- In some studies, high blood pressure was more common when people were taking leflunomide; have your blood pressure checked from time to time.

Side Effects

Leflunomide is a safe and effective drug for RA that most people can take without problems. Because it is new, there is not much information available about the long-term safety of leflunomide.

Common: There are some relatively common bothersome but not serious side effects such as diarrhea and rash. Most people who take leflunomide notice that their bowel movements become a little looser and more frequent; in some people this becomes a problem and they have diarrhea. GI problems such as nausea and, very occasionally, vomiting sometimes occur. Mild changes in liver enzyme tests are common, and your dose of leflunomide may need to be decreased if that happens.

Less common: A few people notice some hair thinning with leflunomide, but this is seldom a cosmetic problem. Interestingly, although leflunomide suppresses your immune system, it does this selectively, and your risks of infection do not seem to be increased.

Interactions with Other Drugs

Other immunosuppressants: All drugs that suppress the immune system increase the risk of side effects such as infection. The more the immune system is suppressed, the higher the risk. High doses of corticosteroids, either alone or with other drugs such as leflunomide, increase the risk of infection.

Live vaccines: Some vaccines are given as a weaker strain of a live virus. These types of vaccines are usually avoided in people taking drugs such as leflunomide that can suppress the immune system.

Rimfampin *(Rifadin):* Blood levels of the active component of leflunomide increase by about 40 percent when these drugs are combined.

Other drugs: There is not much information available about interactions between leflunomide and other commonly used drugs.

Important Information

- Avoid becoming pregnant while you are taking leflunomide. If you are taking or have taken leflunomide and you want to become pregnant, you should speak to your doctor. You will need to take a course of cholestyramine before you try to become pregnant. After you have taken a course of cholestyramine, a blood test is done to confirm that your blood levels of leflunomide are low before you try to become pregnant.
- Do not take more than the prescribed dose of leflunomide. Leflunomide is not a painkiller. Extra doses will not help when you are hurting, and they may be dangerous.
- Regular monitoring of your liver function tests is important. Two liver enzymes that are checked in people taking leflunomide are the AST (aspartate aminotransferase) and the ALT (alanine aminotransferase).
- Avoid immunizations, except for influenza and pneumonia immunization, unless discussed with your physician.
- Contact your doctor if you develop any serious or prolonged infection or fever.

Common Dose Sizes

Tablets: 10 mg and 20 mg.

Usual Adult Doses

Leflunomide is usually started with a big dose of 100 mg a day for three days. This is to "load" your body with the drug when you start taking it. After that, the usual maintenance dose of leflunomide is 20 mg a day. For some people 10 mg a day works almost as well as 20 mg a day. So if someone is having GI problems such as diarrhea, I try a lower dose—usually 20 mg every second day (equivalent to 10 mg a day). Leflunomide stays in your body for so long that even if you take it every second day, the levels in your body stay high on the day that you are not taking it.

Comments

Leflunomide is one of the newer DMARDs that have improved our choices for treating RA. It is about as effective as methotrexate, which makes it one of the more effective DMARDs for RA. Liver function tests, particularly the AST and ALT, can increase a small amount in some people taking leflunomide. This can usually be controlled by decreasing the dose of leflunomide. Unlike methotrexate, leflunomide has not caused liver scarring, but until we have more long-term information, we won't know exactly how safe it is.

Leflunomide does not work quickly, and it could be anywhere from four to eight weeks, or sometimes longer, before you notice improvement in your RA. Leflunomide is usually prescribed as a single DMARD. There is very little information about using it in combination with other DMARDs. A study showed that leflunomide combined with methotrexate was more effective than methotrexate alone. Unfortunately, abnormal liver function tests were also more common, and there is no long-term information about the safety of leflunomide plus methotrexate combination treatment.

Very preliminary reports show that leflunomide may be helpful for some people with psoriatic arthritis and also to keep vasculitis in remission. When more studies are done, we will know exactly where leflunomide fits in the treatment plan for these problems.

LODINE (SEE ETODOLAC)

LORTAB (SEE ACETAMINOPHEN + NARCOTICS)

MAGNESIUM CHOLINE SALICYLATE (SEE CHOLINE MAGNESIUM SALICYLATE)

MAPROTILINE *(LUDIOMIL)* (see ***PROFILES OF COMMON ANTIDEPRESSANT DRUGS*** UNDER AMITRIPTYLINE)

MECLOFENAMATE SODIUM

Brand Name

Meclomen.

Drug Family

Meclofenamate is a nonsteroidal anti-inflammatory drug (NSAID). There are two big groups of NSAIDs, divided by whether they inhibit both cyclo-oxygenase (COX) enzymes, COX-1 and COX-2, or are more selective for COX-2. Meclofenamate inhibits both COX-1 and COX-2.

Families of Arthritis Problems Prescribed For

NSAIDs are used to treat all kinds of pain and inflammation, whether they affect the joints or not. NSAIDs are used to treat many kinds of arthritis problems, such as RA, gout, ankylosing spondylitis, osteoarthritis, and bursitis. NSAIDs decrease pain and inflammation but they do not change the progression of arthritis.

How It Works

Most NSAIDs inhibit the enzymes COX-1 and COX-2. Inhibiting these cyclo-oxygenase enzymes decreases the formation of chemicals called prostaglandins. Decreasing the prostaglandins made by COX-2 is anti-inflammatory, which is usually why we use NSAIDs. Inhibiting COX-1 makes platelets in your blood less sticky, which is why aspirin is used to treat heart attacks. COX-1 also protects the stomach from ulcers, and blocking COX-1 may be why the risk of peptic ulcers is increased with many NSAIDs.

Avoid

Do not take meclofenamate if you are allergic to it. People who have had a serious allergic reaction (swelling of the face and tongue, and wheezing) to one NSAID can have the same reaction to other NSAIDs. People with asthma or nasal polyps are more likely to be allergic to NSAIDs. NSAIDs are avoided if someone has an active peptic ulcer, is bleeding, or is pregnant.

Take Precautions

- NSAIDs can cause fluid retention and can worsen heart failure and high blood pressure.
- Some people are at higher risk for peptic ulcers caused by NSAIDs. Risk factors are being older than 65 years, having had a previous peptic ulcer, having had a previous bleeding ulcer, and taking a corticosteroid. In people at higher risk for peptic ulcers caused by NSAIDs, most rheumatologists would avoid an NSAID, if possible. If this is not possible, prescribing misoprostol (see MISOPROSTOL—*Cytotec*) or a proton pump inhibitor (see OMEPRAZOLE—*Prilosec*) to protect against peptic ulcers caused by NSAIDs is an option. Another option is to use a COX-2 selective NSAID (see CELECOXIB—*Celebrex* and ROFECOXIB—*Vioxx*). None of these choices is foolproof, and peptic ulcers can still happen.

• NSAIDs have to be used carefully in people who have asthma, a bleeding problem, or liver or kidney problems.

• If you are taking NSAIDs regularly, blood tests will be done from time to time to check your blood count (in case you are losing blood slowly from an ulcer that you may not know about), your creatinine (for kidney function), and liver enzymes. People taking diuretics ("water pills") or ACE (angiotensin converting enzyme) inhibitors—a family of drugs that lowers blood pressure—and people with diabetes, heart failure, or existing kidney problems are more likely to have kidney problems caused by NSAIDs. These people may need more frequent blood tests to check their kidney function.

Side Effects

See NSAIDs.

Interactions with Other Drugs

See NSAIDs.

Important Information

• Taking NSAIDs with food is a good idea and may protect you from indigestion, but it does not prevent peptic ulcers.

• To minimize your GI risks, use the lowest effective dose of an NSAID.

• One of the signs that you may be bleeding from the stomach is if you have pitch-black bowel movements. Bowel movements with altered blood, in addition to being black, are also often runny and very smelly. If this happens, contact your doctor immediately.

Common Dose Sizes

Capsule: 50 mg, 100 mg.

Usual Adult Doses.
The usual adult dose of meclofenamate is 50 or 100 mg taken three or four times a day up to a maximum of 400 mg a day.

Comments
See NSAIDs.

MECLOMEN (SEE MECLOFENAMATE SODIUM)

MELOXICAM

Brand Name
Mobic

Drug Family
Meloxicam is a nonsteroidal anti-inflammatory drug (NSAID). There are two big groups of NSAIDs, divided by whether they inhibit both cyclo-oxygenase (COX) enzymes, COX-1 and COX-2, or are more selective for COX-2. Meloxicam inhibits both COX-1 and COX-2 but is partially selective for COX-2.

Families of Arthritis Problems Prescribed For
NSAIDs are used to treat all kinds of pain and inflammation, whether they affect the joints or not. NSAIDs are used to treat many kinds of arthritis problems, such as RA, osteoarthritis and bursitis. NSAIDs decrease pain and inflammation, but they do not change the progression of arthritis.

How It Works
Most NSAIDs inhibit the enzymes COX-1 and COX-2. Inhibiting these cyclo-oxygenase enzymes decreases the formation of chemicals called prostaglandins. Decreasing the

prostaglandins made by COX-2 is anti-inflammatory, which is usually why we use NSAIDs. Inhibiting COX-1 makes platelets in your blood less sticky, which is why aspirin is used to prevent heart attacks. COX-1 also protects the stomach from ulcers, and blocking COX-1 may be why the risk of peptic ulcers is increased with many NSAIDs. Because meloxicam tends more toward a COX-2 blocking effect it may be kinder on the stomach than nonselective NSAIDs.

Avoid

Do not take meloxicam if you are allergic to it. People who have had a serious allergic reaction (swelling of the face and tongue, and wheezing) to one NSAID can have the same reaction with others. People with asthma or nasal polyps are more likely to be allergic to NSAIDs. NSAIDs are avoided if someone has an active peptic ulcer, is bleeding or is pregnant.

Take Precautions

- NSAIDs can cause fluid retention and can worsen heart failure and high blood pressure.
- Some people have a higher risk for peptic ulcers caused by NSAIDs. Risk factors are being older than 65 years, having had a previous peptic ulcer, having had a previous bleeding ulcer, and taking a corticosteroid. In people at higher risk for peptic ulcers caused by NSAIDs, most rheumatologists would avoid an NSAID, if possible. If this is not possible, then prescribing misoprostol (see MISOPROSTOL—*Cytotec*) or a proton pump inhibitor (see OMEPRAZOLE—*Prilosec*) to protect against peptic ulcers caused by NSAIDs is an option. Another option is to use a COX-2 selective NSAID (see CELECOXIB—*Celebrex* and ROFECOXIB—*Vioxx*). None of these choices is foolproof, and peptic ulcers can still develop.

• NSAIDs have to be used carefully in people who have asthma, a bleeding problem, or liver or kidney problems.

• If you are taking NSAIDs regularly, blood tests will be done from time to time to check your blood count (in case you are losing blood slowly from an ulcer that you may not know about), your creatinine (for kidney function), and liver enzymes. People taking diuretics ("water pills") or ACE inhibitors (angiotensin converting enzyme inhibitors—a family of drugs that lowers blood pressure) and people with diabetes, heart failure or existing kidney problems are more likely to have kidney problems caused by NSAIDs. These people may need more frequent blood tests to check their kidney function.

Side Effects

See NSAIDs.

Meloxicam is one of the NSAIDs partially selective for COX-2 and may cause less GI problems than nonselective NSAIDs.

Interactions with Other Drugs

See NSAIDs.

Important Information

• Taking NSAIDs with food is a good idea and may protect you from indigestion, but it does not prevent peptic ulcers.

• To minimize your GI risks use the lowest effective dose of an NSAID.

• One of the signs that you may be bleeding from the stomach is if you have pitch-black bowel movements. Bowel movements with altered blood, in addition to being black, are also often runny and very smelly. If this happens contact your doctor immediately.

Common Dose Sizes

Tablet : 7.5 mg.

Usual Adult Doses

The usual adult dose of meloxicam is 7.5 mg a day. The maximum daily dose is 15 mg.

Comments

See NSAIDs.

There is some information suggesting that meloxicam causes less GI problems than nonselective NSAIDs but we do not know how it compares with the COX-2 selective NSAIDs.

MEPERIDINE

Brand Name

Demerol.

Sometimes Called

Meperidine hydrochloride, Pethidine.

Drug Family

Meperidine is a strong narcotic analgesic (painkiller).

Families of Arthritis Problems Prescribed For

Meperidine is used for severe uncontrolled pain. Strong narcotic analgesics are usually prescribed only for pain that is not controlled by acetaminophen alone, or an NSAID alone, or weaker narcotics such as codeine or hydrocodone. Narcotics do not affect inflammation.

How It Works

Narcotics decrease pain by acting through specific receptors in the brain.

Avoid

Do not take meperidine if you are allergic to it. Real allergic reactions are rare, but a lot of people get side effects, such as nausea or feeling "spacy," from narcotics. Avoid meperidine if you have had an addiction problem. Do not take meperidine if you are taking, or have recently taken, a monoamine oxidase inhibitor antidepressant (See Interactions with Other Drugs.)

Take Precautions

- Do not drink alcohol while you are taking narcotics.
- There is a risk of becoming addicted to narcotics. Use narcotics only for pain, not to feel good. If possible, limit the dose and how long you take them. One physician should be responsible for all your narcotic prescriptions.
- Caution is needed in the elderly and in people with poor liver, lung, or kidney function.
- In people with poor kidney function, one of the breakdown products of meperidine can accumulate and cause seizures.

Side Effects

Strong narcotics often cause minor side effects. People vary in how they respond to different narcotics.

Common: Nausea, vomiting, constipation, poor appetite, dizziness, lightheadedness or feeling "spacy," sleepiness, low blood pressure, and a slow heart rate are common.

Less common: An allergy with rash, hives, or asthma can occur. Confusion, feeling nervous or agitated, sleeping badly, feeling "high," becoming addicted and trying to get higher doses of narcotic to feel good rather than to control pain are occasionally problems. Too high a dose of meperidine can suppress the drive to breathe.

Interactions with Other Drugs

Any other sedative drug: Narcotics make people sleepy, and an overdose can make people unconscious. Combining a narcotic with another sedative drug, such as alcohol, is dangerous.

Monoamine oxidase inhibitor antidepressants Isocarboxazid *(Marplan),* phenelzine *(Nardil),* and tranylcypromine *(Parnate):* There is a risk of serious heart and blood pressure side effects, and even death, if these drugs are combined with meperidine.

Selegiline *(Eldepryl):* Selegiline is a drug used to treat Parkinson's disease. The combination of selegiline with meperidine has caused serious side effects.

Serotonin uptake inhibitors: Fluoxetine *(Prozac)* and other selective serotonin re-uptake inhibitor antidepressants are usually avoided because they increase the risk of serious side effects.

Cimetidine: The blood levels of meperidine can be increased by cimetidine.

Important Information

- Don't take more than the prescribed dose.
- Don't drink alcohol while you are taking narcotic painkillers.
- Narcotics may cause drowsiness and affect your concentration for driving and other tasks.
- Meperidine is a narcotic and can be addictive (see Comments).
- Narcotics are dangerous in overdose and must be kept away from children.

Common Dose Sizes

Tablets: 50 mg, 100 mg.
Injection: various preparations.

Usual Adult Doses

To control acute pain in adults, the usual starting dose of meperidine is 50 mg to 150 mg taken every three to four hours.

Comments

Meperidine is not suitable for long-term use because it has a breakdown product that can cause seizures.

There is some controversy about how narcotic analgesics should be used to control chronic "benign" pain, meaning chronic pain not caused by cancer. This is particularly true of the strong narcotics such as morphine and meperidine. Some physicians think that the risk of addiction and abuse is too high and do not use strong narcotics for any type of arthritis pain. Others limit narcotic prescriptions to short periods, such as a few days. Others prescribe strong narcotics only when devastating arthritis problems are causing severe pain that cannot be controlled by other treatments. Most rheumatologists do not use strong narcotics for fibromyalgia or chronic lower back pain.

A clue to addictive behavior is if you are trying to get bigger doses of the drug and are not really using the bigger doses to control pain. The risk of addiction is higher in people who themselves, or whose family members, have had an addiction problem (alcohol or drugs). I have a few rules for my patients about narcotic prescriptions.

1. Use narcotics only for pain, not to feel good.
2. If you don't have pain, don't take them.
3. Get all your narcotic prescriptions from one doctor and from one pharmacy.
4. Escalating the dose can be an early sign of a problem.
5. Never sell, swap, or hoard narcotics.

6. If you are in the position of wanting to fool doctors or do illegal things such as forging signatures to get narcotic prescriptions, things are way out of control and you need to speak with your physician about getting help.

MESNA

Brand Name
Mesnex.

Drug Family
Mesna binds to one of the toxic breakdown products of cyclophosphamide (*Cytoxan*) in the urine.

Families of Arthritis Problems Prescribed For
Mesna is used to prevent bladder irritation in people being treated with intravenous cyclophosphamide (*Cytoxan*).

How It Works
Mesna has no effect on vasculitis or arthritis problems but works by binding to the toxic breakdown products of cyclophosphamide (*Cytoxan*), making them less toxic to the bladder.

Avoid
Do not take Mesna if you are allergic to it.

Side Effects

Common: Mesna often causes a bad taste in the mouth. It can also cause headache, diarrhea, nausea, and muscle pain.

Less common: An allergic rash or hives.

Common Dose Sizes

Mesna comes only in a 100 mg per ml preparation that is made for injection. Some physicians also give this preparation by mouth (see Usual Adult Doses).

Usual Adult Doses

The total dose of mesna usually depends on your dose of cyclophosphamide. The dose of mesna is usually more than the dose of cyclophosphamide. Someone who receives 500 mg of cyclophosphamide might also receive 500 to 1,000 mg of mesna. Mesna is usually divided into several doses and is given approximately every three hours during and for up to twelve hours after the cyclophosphamide infusion. Most physicians give the first one or two doses of mesna intravenously. It is diluted in a bag of saline and given slowly. After someone has finished his or her cyclophosphamide infusion and gone home, it is sometimes convenient to give the last dose or two of mesna by mouth. To do this the mesna is diluted in a soda drink or in apple or orange juice.

Comments

Some rheumatologists use mesna when they prescribe monthly IV cyclophosphamide. The risk of bladder problems is very low with monthly IV cyclophosphamide. Bladder problems are more common when cyclophosphamide is given as tablets that you have to take every day (see CYCLOPHOSPHAMIDE). Mesna is short-acting, and it is not practical to use it to protect the bladder against cyclophosphamide tablets that you take every day.

METHOCARBAMOL

Brand Names

Delaxin, Marbaxin, Robaxin, Robomol.

Drug Family

Methocarbamol is a muscle relaxer.

Families of Arthritis Problems Prescribed For

Methocarbamol is often used to treat painful muscle spasms but is also useful for some people with fibromyalgia.

How It Works

We do not know exactly how methocarbamol works, but it probably decreases the nerve signals to muscles.

Avoid

Do not take methocarbamol if you are allergic to it.

Take Precautions

• Caution is needed in people with poor liver or kidney function or people who have had seizures.

Side Effects

Common: Drowsiness or dizziness.

Less common: Flushing, nausea, and rash.

Rare: Allergic reactions and bone-marrow problems.

Interactions with Other Drugs

Any other sedative drug: Methocarbamol can make people sleepy, so combining it with any other sedative drug, such as alcohol, can be dangerous.

Important Information

• Don't take more than the prescribed dose.

• Don't drink alcohol while you are taking methocarbamol.

• Methocarbamol can cause drowsiness and affect your concentration for driving and other tasks.

Common Dose Sizes

Tablets: 500 mg, 750 mg.

Usual Adult Doses

The usual dose of methocarbamol in adults who have a problem for only a day or two is 500 mg to 1 g taken two to four times a day. For fibromyalgia a single dose of 500 mg to 1 g at night is often used.

Comments

The sedative effect of methocarbamol is sometimes helpful to improve sleep in fibromyalgia. A muscle relaxer treats symptoms. If it doesn't help you, there is no point in taking it.

METHOTREXATE

Brand Names

Folex, Rheumatrex.

Sometimes Called

MTX.

Drug Family

Methotrexate is an anticancer drug that in low doses modulates the immune system. Methotrexate was first used to treat cancer and was then found to be useful for treating some rheumatic problems. Much smaller doses of methotrexate are used to treat rheumatic problems than are used to treat cancer. Side effects are much less common with these lower doses than with cancer chemotherapy doses.

Families of Arthritis Problems Prescribed For

Methotrexate is one of the most effective disease-modifying antirheumatic drugs (DMARDs) available and is used to treat rheumatoid arthritis and psoriatic arthritis. It is also sometimes used to treat systemic lupus erythematosus, dermatomyositis, or polymyositis and other connective-tissue problems. Methotrexate is sometimes used as "maintenance" treatment to hold vasculitis in remission. In people who need high doses of corticosteroids to control a rheumatic problem, starting treatment with methotrexate often means that the dose of corticosteroid can be decreased. In this situation methotrexate is acting as a "steroid-sparing" agent.

How It Works

Methotrexate blocks an enzyme, dihydrofolate reductase, that is important in making the active form of the vitamin folic acid. Blocking the synthesis of folic acid explains the anticancer effects of methotrexate, but this is probably not the way methotrexate works in arthritis problems. Methotrexate has many other effects that might explain how it works. One of these is that it increases the release of a chemical called adenosine.

Avoid

Do not take methotrexate if you are allergic to it. People who have liver problems or poor kidney function should not take methotrexate. Methotrexate is avoided in pregnancy. Most rheumatologists would avoid using methotrexate in people who have HIV, hepatitis B, or hepatitis C infection and in people who drink alcohol regularly.

Take Precautions

- Caution is needed in people with decreased liver or kidney function.
- Blood tests will be done to check your blood count, creatinine (a measure of kidney function), and liver function, usually every four to eight weeks.

• Because methotrexate can suppress your immune system, you should take seriously any infections that you may get and have them treated early.

• Methotrexate can harm an unborn baby. Make sure that you are not pregnant before you start taking methotrexate; use reliable contraception while you are taking methotrexate and for a few months after you stop it. Men should not conceive children while taking methotrexate and for a few months after stopping it.

• Do not drink alcohol if you are taking methotrexate. Doing so increases the risks of liver damage.

Side Effects

Methotrexate, in the doses used for arthritis problems, does not often cause serious side effects, and it is one of the most widely used DMARDs for RA.

Common: Methotrexate has some relatively common bothersome but not serious side effects such as mouth ulcers and nausea. These seem to be more of a problem soon after starting methotrexate. Some people can have GI problems such as nausea and, very occasionally, vomiting soon after they have taken their weekly dose of methotrexate. Mild changes in liver enzyme tests are common, and your dose of methotrexate may need to be decreased if that happens.

Less common: Methotrexate can sometimes make rheumatoid nodules, small bumps on the elbows and fingers, worse. Some people find that methotrexate makes them feel more fatigued than usual, particularly on the day of their weekly dose. If you take methotrexate, stay out of the sun because it can increase your sensitivity to sunlight. A few people have some hair thinning with methotrexate, but this very seldom causes cosmetic problems.

Rare: Methotrexate can cause a lung problem, similar to pneumonia, called "methotrexate lung." This problem can look much like pneumonia and cause cough, fever, shortness of breath, and an abnormal chest X-ray. The problem usually gets better when methotrexate is stopped, but it can be very serious. Methotrexate lung can come back if someone who has had the problem recovers and then starts methotrexate again, but it does not come back in everyone. It is difficult to diagnose methotrexate lung because there is no definite test for it. This means that it is difficult to be sure how often methotrexate lung happens. Most experts think that the risk is about one out of a hundred. People who smoke or who already have lung problems may have a higher risk for lung problems with methotrexate.

Irreversible liver scarring is rare but serious. The risk is low and is estimated to be about one in 10,000. The risk of methotrexate causing liver problems is higher in people who have had liver problems before (such as from heavy alcohol use or hepatitis) and in people who drink alcohol while on methotrexate. It is rare for methotrexate to depress the bone marrow that makes your blood cells, but it can happen. Methotrexate may increase the risk of infections and certain cancers. This risk is small.

Interactions with Other Drugs

Other immunosuppressants: All drugs that suppress the immune system increase the risk of side effects such as infection. The more the immune system is suppressed, the higher the risk. High doses of corticosteroids, alone or with other drugs such as methotrexate, increase the risk of infection.

Live vaccines: Some vaccines are given as a weaker strain of a live virus. These types of vaccines are usually avoided in people taking drugs that can suppress the immune system.

Trimethoprim: Like methotrexate, trimethoprim blocks the formation of folic acid. Trimethoprim can increase the side effects of methotrexate. We usually try to avoid trimethoprim and antibiotics that contain it, such as cotrimoxazole (*Bactrim, Cotrim, Septra*) in people who are taking methotrexate.

NSAIDs: Aspirin and other NSAIDs can increase the concentrations of methotrexate, usually only by a small amount. In rheumatology practice, with the low doses of methotrexate used, this interaction is seldom important, and methotrexate is often prescribed for RA with an NSAID.

Important Information

- Avoid becoming pregnant while you are taking methotrexate and for a couple of months after stopping it.
- Take methotrexate only once a week.
- Do not take more than the prescribed dose of methotrexate. Methotrexate is not a painkiller. Extra doses will not help when you are hurting and may be very dangerous.
- Regular monitoring of your blood count and liver function tests is important. Two liver enzymes that are checked in people taking methotrexate are the AST (Aspartate aminotransferase) and the ALT (Alanine aminotransferase).
- Avoid immunizations, except for influenza and pneumonia, unless discussed with your physician.
- Contact your doctor if you develop any serious or prolonged infection or fever.
- Remember that methotrexate lung can mimic pneumonia. So if you develop pneumonia, particularly if it does not seem to be responding to treatment, stop your methotrexate and remind any physicians looking after you that you are taking methotrexate and that it can cause a lung problem that can look like pneumonia. This does not mean that you have to panic every time you get a sniffly nose or a bit of a cough—something that happens to most of us several times a year.

Common Dose Sizes

Tablets: Methotrexate comes in 2.5 mg tablets. These tablets are also available as packs that have common weekly doses prepacked on cards with two, three, four, five, or six tablets. Injection: 25 mg/ml (2 ml vial) and other strengths.

Usual Adult Doses

Methotrexate comes in 2.5 mg tablets. The usual dose of methotrexate is given in a once-a-week dose of between three and six tablets. This means that most people's weekly intake is between 7.5 and 15 mg. Higher doses are occasionally used in RA (up to 25 mg a week) because in some people higher doses control the arthritis better. Methotrexate in doses higher than 15 mg a week is often given by a subcutaneous (under the skin) injection because the absorption is better. Most people can learn how to give themselves a weekly injection without a problem, or else a relative or friend can learn how to do it.

Comments

Methotrexate has revolutionized the treatment of RA. It was the first treatment of RA that helped most people who took it, and most people could take it for long periods.

When people talk of methotrexate as "anticancer treatment," they are often not accurate. The way methotrexate is used to treat rheumatic problems is very different from the way it is used to treat cancer, and calling methotrexate "chemo" does it an injustice. The side effects of methotrexate can sound scary. But remember that methotrexate is one of the most widely-used DMARDs. We have a lot of experience using methotrexate, and on average it is a safe drug. Remember that your risks are not high and can be decreased by not drinking alcohol and by having regular blood checks.

Also remember that if rheumatoid arthritis is not effectively treated, it can be a serious problem for some people.

Liver function tests, particularly the AST and ALT, can increase a small amount in some people taking methotrexate. This can usually be taken care of by decreasing the dose of methotrexate. Because NSAIDs can also sometimes increase the liver enzymes, we sometimes try and stop NSAIDs if someone who is taking methotrexate has had an increase in his liver function tests. In people who have abnormal liver enzymes that do not come down after the dose of methotrexate is decreased, methotrexate is stopped, or else a liver biopsy is done to make sure that methotrexate is not damaging the liver. Most people with arthritis-related problems who are taking methotrexate do not need a liver biopsy as part of routine monitoring. But in people with psoriasis who take methotrexate, because they seem to be more sensitive to methotrexate liver damage, most rheumatologists recommend that a liver biopsy should be done every few years.

Set aside one day of the week as your methotrexate day. If you are nauseated by methotrexate, it can help to split your weekly dose into two doses and take them twelve hours apart. Folic acid supplements (1 mg a day) decrease some of the side effects of methotrexate, and many rheumatologists prescribe them routinely (see FOLIC ACID). The injectable form of methotrexate is much cheaper than the tablets. It is exactly the same drug. To save their patients money, some physicians prescribe the injectable form of methotrexate to be taken by mouth. These people take their weekly dose of methotrexate by diluting the appropriate dose of the injectable methotrexate preparation in fruit juice and drinking it.

Methotrexate is still one of the most effective DMARDs available to control RA. It does not work quickly, and it could be anywhere between four and twelve weeks before you notice improvement. Methotrexate is often prescribed as a single DMARD initially, but if your RA is not controlled, a combination treatment is often tried. Studies of methotrexate combined with cyclosporine or infliximab, or methotrexate combined with sulfasalazine and hydroxychloroquine, have shown that these combinations can be helpful for some people who still have active RA on methotrexate.

Methotrexate is usually not the first drug used to try to get most types of vasculitis into remission. But with problems such as Wegener's granulomatosis, methotrexate is sometimes used to hold remission after cyclophosphamide has controlled the problem.

MIACALCIN (SEE CALCITONIN)

MINOCYCLINE

Brand Name
Minocin.

Sometimes Called
Minocycline hydrochloride.

Drug Family
Minocycline is a tetracycline antibiotic.

Families of Arthritis Problems Prescribed For
Minocycline is used as a disease-modifying antirheumatic drug (DMARD) to treat rheumatoid arthritis. In clinical practice it is more often used to treat acne.

How It Works
We do not know how minocycline works in RA. It is prob-

ably working in ways that are not related to its antibiotic actions.

Avoid

Do not take minocycline if you are allergic to it. Minocycline is avoided in pregnancy and is not used in children.

Take Precautions

- Caution is needed in people with poor kidney function.

Side Effects

Common: Diarrhea, nausea, and increased skin sensitivity to sunlight are fairly common. Dizziness is less common. Tetracyclines are avoided in children because they cause discoloration of the permanent teeth.

Rare: A rash, which can cause darkening of patches of skin, or allergic reactions are uncommon. There is a type of lupus called "drug-induced lupus," which minocycline can rarely cause. This type of lupus goes away when minocycline is stopped.

Interactions with Other Drugs

Antacids: The absorption of minocycline is decreased if you take it with antacids.

Oral contraceptives: Minocycline can decrease the effectiveness of oral contraceptives.

Important Information

- Minocycline can increase the sensitivity of your skin to sunlight, and you may develop a rash or sunburn more easily than usual.
- Do not take minocycline with antacids or milk because it will be poorly absorbed.

Common Dose Sizes

Capsule: 100 mg.

Usual Adult Doses

The usual adult dose of minocycline in RA is 100 mg twice a day.

Comments

Minocycline has received a lot of positive press. Books have been written describing it as a wonder drug and a cure for all types of arthritis problems. Unfortunately, this is not true. Minocycline is modestly effective in RA but, on average, it is not as effective as stronger DMARDs such as methotrexate, for example. I place minocycline on about the same level as hydroxychloroquine. The response to minocycline, as is true for all DMARDs, is much more impressive when it is used early in the development of RA. I occasionally use minocycline in people with early and mild RA, particularly if they cannot take other DMARDs. There is a very preliminary report of minocycline improving the skin elasticity in people with scleroderma. This has led to minocycline being prescribed for some people with scleroderma. There is not enough information available to decide whether minocycline is an effective treatment for scleroderma. If my patients with scleroderma request minocycline, I discuss the risks and benefits and we decide which treatment is best.

Minocycline is more expensive and tends to have more side effects than other tetracyclines, such as doxycycline. Some rheumatologists prescribe doxycycline and minocycline interchangeably. I do not know if doxycycline and minocycline are equally effective in RA. The biggest studies were done with minocycline, so the evidence supports it.

MISOPROSTOL

Brand Name
Cytotec.

Sometimes Called
Prostaglandin analog.

Drug Family
Misoprostol belongs to the family of drugs that protects the stomach against peptic ulcers caused by NSAIDs. It is a prostaglandin-like chemical that has been designed to replace the prostaglandins that protect your stomach.

Families of Arthritis Problems Prescribed For
Misoprostol does not treat arthritis. It is taken to protect your stomach against the gastrointestinal side effects that can be caused by nonsteroidal anti-inflammatory drugs.

How It Works
NSAIDs, particularly the nonselective ones that inhibit both cyclo-oxygenase (COX) enzymes—COX-1 and COX-2—decrease the formation of prostaglandins that protect your stomach. Misoprostol acts as a prostaglandin replacement.

Avoid
Misoprostol causes abnormalities of the unborn baby and can cause abortion. Do not take misoprostol if you are pregnant or if there is any possibility that you may become pregnant. Do not take misoprostol if you are allergic to it.

Take Precautions

• Misoprostol is damaging to the unborn baby. Make sure that you are not pregnant before you start misoprostol. Use reliable contraception while you are taking it.

• I find it more convenient to avoid misoprostol in women who could become pregnant and to use an alternative type of GI protection in them.

Side Effects

Common: The most common side effects of misoprostol are diarrhea and stomach cramps. Most people have slightly loose stools with misoprostol, but this is not usually a problem. In fact, it can be useful for some people who are usually constipated. With higher doses of misoprostol, diarrhea can be a problem.

Less common: Nausea, vomiting, headache, and vaginal bleeding are less common.

Interactions with Other Drugs

There are no important drug interactions with misoprostol.

Important Information

• Do not become pregnant while you are taking misoprostol.

• Misoprostol can cause loose stools and diarrhea.

• Misoprostol needs to be taken regularly to prevent the GI problems caused by NSAIDs. It will not protect you if you take it only when you are having GI problems.

Common Dose Sizes

Tablets: 100 micrograms (mcg), 200 micrograms.

Usual Adult Doses

The usual adult dose of misoprostol to protect against GI problems caused by NSAIDs is 100 to 200 mcg four times a day. The 200 mcg four times a day dose schedule is most effective for preventing GI problems, but with this dose, most people have trouble remembering to take it or have loose stools. In clinical practice, lower doses such as 200 mcg two or three times a day are often used.

Comments

Misoprostol cuts the risk of serious GI problems in people taking nonselective NSAIDs by about half. Nonselective NSAIDs are a relatively common cause of serious GI problems, particularly in people at high risk. Risk factors are being older than 65 years, having had a previous peptic ulcer, having had a previous bleeding ulcer, and taking a corticosteroid. In people at higher risk for peptic ulcers caused by NSAIDs, most rheumatologists would avoid an NSAID, if possible. If this is not possible, prescribing misoprostol or a proton pump inhibitor (see OMEPRAZOLE—*Prilosec*) to protect against peptic ulcers caused by NSAIDs is an option. Another option is to use COX-2 selective NSAIDs (see CELECOXIB—*Celebrex* and ROFECOXIB—*Vioxx*), which are kinder on the stomach.

None of these choices is foolproof, and peptic ulcers can still happen. There are many unanswered questions about protecting against GI problems caused by NSAIDs. Do the serious ulcer problems caused by older, nonselective NSAIDs in relatively few people mean that everyone should be treated with a new COX-2 selective NSAID, although it may cost more? Are there side effects from the new COX-2 inhibitor NSAIDs that we don't know about yet? In people at higher risk for peptic ulcers, are COX-2 selective NSAIDs safer than a nonselective NSAID taken with a stomach protective agent such as misoprostol? We don't know the answers to these questions. Most rheumatologists do not use GI protection in every person because in people at low risk it is not cost-effective. My approach is not to change people who are stable on their older NSAID to a newer COX-2 selective drug. In people at higher risk for NSAID ulcer problems, I discuss the choices available and either use a COX-2 selective drug, or an older NSAID with either misoprostol (see MISOPROSTOL—*Cytotec*) or a proton pump inhibitor (see OMEPRAZOLE—*Prilosec*) to protect against ulcers. As more information becomes available, we will have clearer answers to these questions.

MOBIC (SEE MELOXICAM)

MOTRIN (SEE IBUPROFEN)

MYCOPHENOLATE MOFETIL

Brand Name
CellCept.

Sometimes Called
Mycophenolic acid.

Drug Family
Mycophenolate modulates the immune system and is an antirejection drug used in people who have received an organ transplant.

Families of Arthritis Problems Prescribed For
Mycophenolate is not approved by the FDA for the treatment of any rheumatic problem. It is being tested as a disease-

modifying antirheumatic drug (DMARD) for RA, but the studies have not been completed. Some rheumatologists are using mycophenolate in people with systemic lupus erythematosus and as "maintenance" treatment in people with vasculitis to hold the problem in remission. In people who need high doses of corticosteroids to control their autoimmune problem, mycophenolate, acting as a "steroid-sparing" agent, may mean that lower doses of corticosteroids can be used.

How It Works

Mycophenolate interferes with DNA formation by blocking the formation of purines (building blocks for DNA), particularly in cells such as lymphocytes, which regulate your immune response.

Avoid

Do not take mycophenolate if you are allergic to it. Mycophenolate is avoided in pregnancy.

Take Precautions

- Caution is needed in people with decreased liver or kidney function.
- Your blood count will be checked from time to time, often every few weeks initially, and then less often once you are on a stable dose of mycophenolate.
- Because mycophenolate suppresses your immune system, you should take seriously any infections that you may get and have them treated early.

Side Effects

Common: Gastrointestinal (GI) symptoms such as vomiting, diarrhea, stomach pain, and nausea are common but not serious.

Less common: Suppression of your bone marrow can cause

a low white blood cell count. Mild changes in liver enzyme tests are uncommon. Shingles (also called herpes zoster), a painful blistering rash caused by reactivation of the chickenpox virus, is more common. Mycophenolate increases the risk of infections. These can be regular infections, such as pneumonia, but can also be less common infections, such as tuberculosis.

Rare: Serious allergic reactions are rare. Mycophenolate may slightly increase the risk of some malignancies, such as lymphoma, leukemia, and skin cancers.

Interactions with Other Drugs

Antacids (*Maalox* and many others): Antacids interfere with the absorption of mycophenolate into your body. If you are taking antacids, do not take them at the same time as your mycophenolate.

Other immunosuppressants: All drugs that suppress the immune system increase the risk of side effects such as infection. The more the immune system is suppressed, the higher the risk. High doses of corticosteroids, alone or with other drugs such as mycophenolate, increase the risk of infection.

Live vaccines: Some vaccines are given as a weaker strain of a live virus. These vaccines are usually avoided in people taking drugs such as mycophenolate that can suppress the immune system.

Probenecid *(Benemid):* Blood levels of mycophenolate are higher in people taking probenecid, and the dose of mycophenolate may need to be reduced.

Important Information

- Avoid becoming pregnant while you are taking mycophenolate.
- Do not take more than the prescribed dose of mycophenolate.

• Regular monitoring of your blood count is important.

• Avoid immunizations, except for influenza and pneumonia, unless discussed with your physician.

• Contact your doctor if you develop any serious or prolonged infection or fever.

Common Dose Sizes

Capsule: 250 mg.

Tablet: 500 mg.

Usual Adult Doses

The usual adult dose of mycophenolate is 1 g twice a day. Sometimes starting at a lower dose and building up cuts down on the nuisance side effects, particularly GI side effects.

Comments

It is not clear what role mycophenolate is going to play in the treatment of arthritis-related problems. It is one of the newer drugs that are being evaluated, and there is very little information available. So far it seems most similar to azathioprine as far as efficacy and side effects go, but it is more expensive. Some rheumatologists are trying mycophenolate as an alternative to drugs such as azathioprine (see AZATHIOPRINE), either if they have not worked or if there have been problems with side effects.

MYOCHRYSINE (SEE GOLD INJECTIONS)

NABUMETONE

Brand Name

Relafen.

Drug Family

Nabumetone is a nonsteroidal anti-inflammatory drug (NSAID). There are two big groups of NSAIDs, divided by whether they inhibit both cyclo-oxygenase (COX) enzymes, COX-1 and COX-2, or are more selective for COX-2. Nabumetone inhibits both COX-1 and COX-2 but may be partially selective for COX-2.

Families of Arthritis Problems Prescribed For

NSAIDs are used to treat all kinds of pain and inflammation, whether they affect the joints or not. NSAIDs are used to treat many kinds of arthritis problems, such as RA, ankylosing spondylitis, osteoarthritis, and bursitis. NSAIDs decrease pain and inflammation, but they do not change the progression of arthritis.

How It Works

Most NSAIDs inhibit the enzymes COX-1 and COX-2. Inhibiting these cyclo-oxygenase enzymes decreases the formation of chemicals called prostaglandins. Decreasing the prostaglandins made by COX-2 is anti-inflammatory, which is usually why we use NSAIDs. Inhibiting COX-1 makes platelets in your blood less sticky, which is why aspirin is used to treat heart attacks. COX-1 also protects the stomach from ulcers, and blocking COX-1 may be why the risk of peptic ulcers is increased with many NSAIDs.

Avoid

Do not take nabumetone if you are allergic to it. People who have had a serious allergic reaction (swelling of the face and tongue, and wheezing) to one NSAID can have the same reaction to others. People with asthma or nasal polyps are more likely to be allergic to NSAIDs. NSAIDs are avoided if someone has an active peptic ulcer, is bleeding, or is pregnant.

Take Precautions

• NSAIDs can cause fluid retention and can worsen heart failure and high blood pressure.

• Some people are at higher risk for peptic ulcers caused by NSAIDs. Risk factors are being older than 65 years, having had a previous peptic ulcer, having had a previous bleeding ulcer, and taking a corticosteroid. In people at higher risk for peptic ulcers caused by NSAIDs, most rheumatologists would avoid an NSAID, if possible. If this is not possible, then prescribing misoprostol (see MISOPROSTOL—*Cytotec*) or a proton pump inhibitor (see OMEPRAZOLE—*Prilosec*) to protect against peptic ulcers caused by NSAIDs is an option. Another option is to use a COX-2 selective NSAID (see CELECOXIB—*Celebrex* and ROFECOXIB—*Vioxx*). None of these choices is foolproof, and peptic ulcers can still happen.

• NSAIDs have to be used carefully in people who have asthma, a bleeding problem, or liver or kidney problems.

• If you are taking NSAIDs regularly, blood tests will be done from time to time to check your blood count (in case you are losing blood slowly from an ulcer that you may not know about), your creatinine (for kidney function), and liver enzymes. People taking diuretics ("water pills") or ACE (angiotensin converting enzyme) inhibitors—a family of drugs that lowers blood pressure—and people with diabetes, heart failure, or existing kidney problems are more likely to have kidney problems caused by NSAIDs. These people may need more frequent blood tests to check their kidney function.

Side Effects

See NSAIDs.

Nabumetone may cause fewer gastrointestinal (GI) side effects than other NSAIDs that are not selective for COX-2.

Interactions with Other Drugs

See NSAIDs.

Important Information

- Taking NSAIDs with food is a good idea and may protect you from indigestion, but it does not prevent peptic ulcers.
- To minimize your GI risks, use the lowest effective dose of an NSAID.
- One of the signs that you may be bleeding from the stomach is if you have pitch-black bowel movements. Bowel movements with altered blood, in addition to being black, are also often runny and very smelly. If this happens, contact your doctor immediately.

Common Dose Sizes

Tablet: 500 mg, 750 mg.

Usual Adult Doses

The usual adult dose of nabumetone is 1,000 mg a day. This can be taken as one dose or split into two doses. The usual maximum dose is a 2,000 mg a day split into two doses.

Comments

See NSAIDs.

There is some information showing that nabumetone may cause fewer GI problems than other commonly used non-selective NSAIDs.

NALFON (SEE FENOPROFEN)

NAPRELAN (SEE NAPROXEN)

NAPROSYN (SEE NAPROXEN)

NAPROXEN

Brand Names

Naproxen: *Aleve, Anaprox, Naprosyn.*

Controlled-release (slow-release) naproxen: *Naprelan*

Sometimes Called

Naproxen sodium.

Drug Family

Naproxen is a nonsteroidal anti-inflammatory drug (NSAID). There are two big groups of NSAIDs, divided by whether they inhibit both cyclo-oxygenase (COX) enzymes, COX-1 and COX-2, or are more selective for COX-2. Naproxen inhibits both COX-1 and COX-2.

Families of Arthritis Problems Prescribed For

NSAIDs are used to treat all kinds of pain and inflammation, whether they affect the joints or not. NSAIDs are used to treat many kinds of arthritis problems, such as RA, gout, ankylosing spondylitis, osteoarthritis, and bursitis. NSAIDs decrease pain and inflammation, but they do not change the progression of arthritis.

How It Works

Most NSAIDs inhibit the enzymes COX-1 and COX-2. Inhibiting these cyclo-oxygenase enzymes decreases the formation of chemicals called prostaglandins. Decreasing the prostaglandins made by COX-2 is anti-inflammatory, which is usually why we use NSAIDs. Inhibiting COX-1 makes

platelets in your blood less sticky, which is why aspirin is used to treat heart attacks. COX-1 also protects the stomach from ulcers, and blocking COX-1 may be why the risk of peptic ulcers is increased with many NSAIDs.

Avoid

Do not take naproxen if you are allergic to it. People who have had a serious allergic reaction (swelling of the face and tongue, and wheezing) to one NSAID can have the same reaction to others. People with asthma or nasal polyps are more likely to be allergic to NSAIDs. NSAIDs are avoided if someone has an active peptic ulcer, is bleeding, or is pregnant.

Take Precautions

- NSAIDs can cause fluid retention and can worsen heart failure and high blood pressure.
- Naproxen can increase your skin's sensitivity to sunlight, and you may develop a rash or sunburn more easily than usual.
- Some people are at higher risk for peptic ulcers caused by NSAIDs. Risk factors are being older than 65 years, having had a previous peptic ulcer, having had a previous bleeding ulcer, and taking a corticosteroid. In people at higher risk for peptic ulcers caused by NSAIDs, most rheumatologists would avoid an NSAID, if possible. If this is not possible, then prescribing misoprostol (see MISOPROSTOL—*Cytotec*) or a proton pump inhibitor (see OMEPRAZOLE—*Prilosec*) to protect against peptic ulcers caused by NSAIDs is an option. Another option is to use a COX-2 selective NSAID (see CELECOXIB—*Celebrex* and ROFECOXIB—*Vioxx*). None of these choices is foolproof, and peptic ulcers can still happen.
- NSAIDs have to be used carefully in people who have asthma, a bleeding problem, or liver or kidney problems.

• If you are taking NSAIDs regularly, blood tests will be done from time to time to check your blood count (in case you are losing blood slowly from an ulcer that you may not know about), your creatinine (for kidney function), and liver enzymes. People taking diuretics ("water pills") or ACE (angiotensin converting enzyme) inhibitors—a family of drugs that lowers blood pressure—and people with diabetes, heart failure, or existing kidney problems are more likely to have kidney problems caused by NSAIDs. These people may need more frequent blood tests to check their kidney function.

Side Effects

See NSAIDs.

Interactions with Other Drugs

See NSAIDs.

Important Information

• Taking NSAIDs with food is a good idea and may protect you from indigestion, but it does not prevent peptic ulcers.

• To minimize your gastrointestinal (GI) risks, use the lowest effective dose of an NSAID.

• One of the signs that you may be bleeding from the stomach is if you have pitch-black bowel movements. Bowel movements with altered blood, in addition to being black, are also often runny and very smelly. If this happens, contact your doctor immediately.

Common Dose Sizes

Tablet: 250 mg, 375 mg, 500 mg.

Sustained-release tablet: 375 mg, 500 mg.

Usual Adult Doses

The usual adult dose of naproxen is 500 mg to 1000 mg a day divided into two doses.

The usual adult starting dose for the controlled-release (slow-release) preparation of naproxen *(Naprelan)* in adults is two 375 mg tablets (750 mg) once a day or two 500 mg tablets (1,000 mg) once a day.

Comments

See NSAIDs.

NEORAL (SEE CYCLOSPORINE)

NEURONTIN (SEE GABAPENTIN)

NITROGLYCERIN OINTMENT

Brand Names

Nitro-Bid Ointment, Nitrol Ointment.

Sometimes Called

Nitropaste.

Drug Family

Nitroglycerin is a vasodilator. It dilates arteries and veins.

Families of Arthritis Problems Prescribed For

Nitroglycerin is most often used to dilate the arteries in the hearts of people who have angina. Nitrogylerin ointment is sometimes used for a particular type of arthritis-related problem called Raynaud's—a problem in which the small blood vessels in the fingers constrict, often in response to cold. Bad Raynaud's, particularly in scleroderma, can cut off the blood supply to the tips of the fingers and they can develop ulcers.

Nitroglycerin paste is sometimes used to improve the blood supply to the fingertips.

How it works

Nitroglycerin dilates blood vessels and improves the blood supply.

Avoid

Do not use nitroglycerin if you are allergic to it. Men taking sildenafil *(Viagra),* a medicine used to improve erections, should not use nitrate or nitroglycerin medicines.

Take Precautions

- Use only small amounts of the ointment on the tips of your fingers.

Side Effects

Common: Nitroglycerin is absorbed from the ointment into your body and dilates blood vessels all over your body. This can cause a flushed feeling, dizziness, and headache.

Interactions with Other Drugs

Sildenafil *(Viagra):* The effects of nitrates, such as nitroglycerin, are increased a lot by sildenafil. People who take sildenafil should not use nitrates because their blood pressure can drop to dangerously low levels.

Common Dose Sizes

Nitroglycerin ointment usually comes as a 2 percent ointment.

Usual Adult Doses

The usual dose in people with heart problems is a 2 cm to 5 cm strip of ointment applied twice a day. For people with fingertip ulcers caused by Raynaud's, much smaller amounts of ointment are applied to the fingertips.

Comments

The use of nitroglycerin paste to treat finger ulcers caused by Raynaud's is not FDA approved, and there is not much information about how effective this treatment is. Fingertip ulcers caused by Raynaud's can be very difficult to control, and different kinds of treatment are often tried. I have not been impressed by the responses to nitroglycerin ointment.

NIZATIDINE (*AXID;* SEE ***PROFILES OF COMMON H_2-RECEPTOR ANTAGONIST DRUGS*** UNDER CIMETIDINE)

NORFLEX (SEE ORPHENADRINE)

NORTRIPTYLINE (*AVENTYL HYDROCHLORIDE, PAMELOR;* SEE ***PROFILES OF COMMON ANTIDEPRESSANT DRUGS*** UNDER AMITRIPTYLINE)

NSAIDs (NONSTEROIDAL ANTI-INFLAMMATORY DRUGS)

Nonselective NSAIDs inhibit both cyclo-oxygenase enzymes (COX-1 and COX-2), have similar good or bad effects, and tend to interact with the same drugs.

Side Effects

Common: NSAIDs are one of the most common medicines we take. Many people tolerate NSAIDs reasonably well. Gastrointestinal (GI) problems, usually indigestion or heartburn, are common reasons why people stop taking NSAIDs.

NSAIDs often cause some fluid retention with a little ankle swelling.

Less common: A serious problem from a peptic ulcer is less common. Peptic ulcers can be silent, without warning symptoms such as indigestion. Small ulcers occur in many people taking NSAIDs without their even knowing it. In people at higher risk (older than 65 years, a previous peptic ulcer, a previous bleeding ulcer, and combined treatment with a corticosteroid), the risk of a serious ulcer problem with nonselective NSAIDs can be as high as three out of every 100 people.

Blood pressure can increase in some people, usually by a small amount. Abnormal liver function tests (usually mild), rashes, ringing in the ears and a feeling of lightheadedness or feeling "spacy" can occur.

Rare: Bleeding from an ulcer, perforation of the bowel, serious liver problems, rash, dizziness, and kidney problems can occur. People who have an allergic reaction to one NSAID and get wheezing, a lumpy and itchy rash, and swelling of the tongue or face are often allergic to other NSAIDs.

Interactions with Other Drugs

Warfarin *(Coumadin):* If possible, NSAIDs are avoided in people taking warfarin or other anticoagulants, because the effects of NSAIDs on platelets increase the risk of bleeding.

NSAIDs: A combination of two NSAIDs is avoided because it does not improve the control of inflammation but does increase the risk of side effects. But if someone on an NSAID needs aspirin to prevent a heart attack or stroke, a low dose of aspirin is often prescribed with the other NSAID.

Methotrexate: Aspirin and other NSAIDs can increase the concentrations of methotrexate, usually only by a small amount. In rheumatology practice, with the low doses of methotrexate used, this interaction is seldom important, and methotrexate is often prescribed for RA with an NSAID.

Lithium: Many NSAIDs can increase lithium levels. Lithium levels are usually monitored, and the dose of lithium can be decreased if needed.

Diuretics ("water pills") or ACE (angiotensin converting enzyme) inhibitors—a family of drugs that lowers blood pressure: Many NSAIDs blunt the ability of these drugs to lower blood pressure.

Comments

Most people take NSAIDs for arthritis pain. There is no convincing evidence that one NSAID is more effective than another for arthritis pain. But people respond differently, and you may find that one particular NSAID suits you much better than the others. There are many NSAIDs on the market. I don't think there is much point in trying a lot of different ones to get greater effect. If two or three NSAIDs don't help much, it usually means that some other type of treatment may be better for you.

Some people with osteoarthritis find that NSAIDs and acetaminophen reduce their pain by about the same amount. If this is the case for you, take acetaminophen because it is safer. Rheumatoid arthritis causes a lot more inflammation than osteoarthritis, and NSAIDs usually control the symptoms of RA better than acetaminophen does. People vary a lot. Some people with RA tell me they find that NSAIDs make very little difference to their symptom control. For them the risks outweigh the benefits, and I suggest that they need not take an NSAID. Other people with RA find that NSAIDs help them a lot, and for them NSAIDs are very useful. RA is virtually never controlled by an NSAID alone, so a disease-modifying antirheumatic drug is introduced early in the treatment plan.

There are many unanswered questions about NSAIDs. Do the serious ulcer problems caused by older nonselective NSAIDs in relatively few people mean that everyone should be treated with a new COX-2 selective NSAID, although it may cost more? Are there side effects from the new COX-2 inhibitor NSAIDs that we don't know about yet? In people at higher risk for peptic ulcers, are COX-2 selective NSAIDs safer than a nonselective NSAID taken with a stomach protective agent such as misoprostol? We don't know the answers to these questions. My approach is not to change people who are stable on their older NSAID to a newer COX-2 selective drug. In people at higher risk for NSAID ulcer problems, I discuss the choices available and either use a COX-2 selective drug or an older NSAID with either misoprostol (see MISOPROSTOL—*Cytotec*) or a proton pump inhibitor (see OMEPRAZOLE—*Prilosec*) to protect against ulcers. As more information becomes available, we will have clearer answers to these questions. I suspect that COX-2 selective NSAIDs, because they are equally effective and are likely to be safer, will replace nonselective NSAIDs as the first choice for most people with arthritis who need NSAIDs.

OMEPRAZOLE

Brand Name

Prilosec.

Drug Family

Omeprazole belongs to a family of drugs that block a "pump" in the stomach that pumps acid into the stomach. This family of drugs is called proton pump inhibitors.

Families of Arthritis Problems Prescribed For

Proton pump inhibitors are not used to treat arthritis, but they are used to treat and prevent peptic ulcers and gastroesophageal reflux disease (GERD)—problems that are common in people who take NSAIDs.

How It Works

Proton pump inhibitors treat and prevent ulcers by decreasing the amount of acid your stomach makes.

Avoid

Do not take proton pump inhibitors if you are allergic to them.

Side Effects

Proton pump inhibitors seldom cause side effects, and most people take them without any problems.

Less common: Constipation, rash, dizziness, diarrhea, back pain, and abdominal pain have been described, but few people have to stop taking a proton pump inhibitor because of these side effects.

Rare: Serious liver, kidney, or bone marrow problems are very rare.

Interactions with Other Drugs

Warfarin *(Coumadin):* Omeprazole increases the anticoagulant (anti–blood clotting) effect of warfarin in some people. If you are taking warfarin to prevent blood clots and start taking omeprazole, you may need to have your blood monitored more frequently than usual, and your dose of warfarin may need to be changed.

Diazepam *(Valium),* Phenytoin *(Dilantin):* Omeprazole can increase the blood levels of these drugs by slowing their breakdown.

Important Information.

- Swallow the capsule whole. Do not chew or crush the granules inside the capsule.
- If you are taking a course of treatment to treat an ulcer, you must finish the prescribed course to make sure your ulcer heals.

Common Dose Sizes

Capsule: 20 mg.

Usual Adult Doses

The usual adult dose of omeprazole to treat duodenal ulcers, to treat GERD, and to prevent ulcers is 20 mg once daily. For active gastric ulcers and bad GERD, higher doses, such as 40 mg a day and sometimes higher, are used.

Comments

Proton pump inhibitors cause few side effects and are effective in treating and preventing ulcers. There is not much to choose between the various drugs available, but there is most information about omeprazole preventing GI problems caused by NSAIDs. On the other hand, lansoprazole and rabeprazole are less likely than omeprazole to interact with other drugs. At first, proton pump inhibitors were used for only short courses of treatment, lasting four to eight weeks because there was a worry that treatment for a long time might cause a type of tumor that was seen in rats treated with high doses of omeprazole for a long time. More experience with proton pump inhibitors has changed our thinking, and many people are on regular treatment for longer periods. The information, so far, is very reassuring, showing no increased risk of cancer with the proton pump inhibitors.

PROFILES OF COMMON PROTON PUMP INHIBITORS

Generic Name	*Brand Name*	*Usual Adult Dose*	*Drug Interactions*
Lansoprazole	*Prevacid*	15 mg to 30 mg a day	+
Omeprazole	*Prilosec*	20 mg to 40 mg a day	++
Rabeprazole	*Aciphex*	20 mg a day	+

OPHTHALMIC SOLUTIONS

(SEE ARTIFICIAL TEARS)

ORPHENADRINE CITRATE

Brand Name

Norflex.

Drug Family

Orphenadrine is a muscle relaxer.

Families of Arthritis Problems Prescribed For

Orphenadrine is used to treat painful muscle spasm.

How It Works

We do not know exactly how orphenadrine works, but it probably decreases the nerve signals to muscles.

Avoid

Do not take orphenadrine if you are allergic to it. Orphenadrine is usually avoided in people with a condition called myasthenia gravis and in people with glaucoma (increased pressure in the eyeball).

Take Precautions

- Caution is needed in people who have heart-rhythm problems.

Side Effects

Common: Drowsiness or dizziness and anticholinergic symptoms such as dry eyes, dry mouth, blurred vision, constipation, and particularly in men with prostate problems, difficulty passing urine can occur.

Less common: Flushing, nausea, and rash.

Interactions with Other Drugs

Any other sedative drug: Orphenadrine can make people sleepy, so combining it with any other sedative drug, such as alcohol, can be dangerous.

Any drug with anticholinergic effects: Combining orphenadrine with another class of drugs that also has anticholinergic side effects, such as antidepressants, will increase the anticholinergic side effects.

Important Information

- Don't take more than the prescribed dose.
- Don't drink alcohol while you are taking orphenadrine.
- Orphenadrine can cause drowsiness and affect your concentration while driving and performing other tasks.

Common Dose Sizes

Tablet: 100 mg.
Sustained-release tablet: 100 mg.

Usual Adult Doses

The usual dose of orphenadrine in adults who have a short-term problem is 100 mg twice a day.

Comments

The sedative effect of orphenadrine is sometimes helpful to improve sleep. A muscle relaxer treats symptoms. If it doesn't help you, there is no point in taking it.

ORUDIS (SEE KETOPROFEN)

ORUVAIL (SEE KETOPROFEN)

OSCAL (SEE CALCIUM)

OXAPROZIN

Brand Name

Daypro.

Drug Family

Oxaprozin is a nonsteroidal anti-inflammatory drug (NSAID). There are two big groups of NSAIDs, divided by whether they inhibit both cyclo-oxygenase (COX) enzymes, COX-1 and COX-2, or are more selective for COX-2. Oxaprozin inhibits both COX-1 and COX-2.

Families of Arthritis Problems Prescribed For

NSAIDs are used to treat all kinds of pain and inflammation, whether they affect the joints or not. NSAIDs are used to treat many kinds of arthritis problems, such as RA, gout, ankylosing spondylitis, osteoarthritis, and bursitis. NSAIDs decrease pain and inflammation, but they do not change the progression of arthritis.

How It Works

Most NSAIDs inhibit the enzymes COX-1 and COX-2. Inhibiting these cyclo-oxygenase enzymes decreases the formation of chemicals called prostaglandins. Decreasing the prostaglandins made by COX-2 is anti-inflammatory, which is usually why we use NSAIDs. Inhibiting COX-1 makes

platelets in your blood less sticky, which is why aspirin is used to treat heart attacks. COX-1 also protects the stomach from ulcers, and blocking COX-1 may be why the risk of peptic ulcers is increased with many NSAIDs.

Avoid

Do not take oxaprozin if you are allergic to it. People who have had a serious allergic reaction (swelling of the face and tongue, and wheezing) to one NSAID can have the same reaction with others. People with asthma or nasal polyps are more likely to be allergic to NSAIDs. NSAIDs are avoided if someone has an active peptic ulcer, is bleeding, or is pregnant.

Take Precautions

- NSAIDs can cause fluid retention and can worsen heart failure and high blood pressure.
- Some people are at higher risk for peptic ulcers caused by NSAIDs. Risk factors are being older than 65 years, having had a previous peptic ulcer, having had a previous bleeding ulcer, and taking a corticosteroid. In people at higher risk for peptic ulcers caused by NSAIDs, most rheumatologists would avoid an NSAID, if possible. If this is not possible, then prescribing misoprostol (see MISOPROSTOL—*Cytotec*) or a proton pump inhibitor (see OMEPRAZOLE—*Prilosec*) to protect against peptic ulcers caused by NSAIDs is an option. Another option is to use a COX-2 selective NSAID (see CELECOXIB—*Celebrex* and ROFECOXIB—*Vioxx*). None of these choices is foolproof, and peptic ulcers can still happen.
- NSAIDs have to be used carefully in people who have asthma, a bleeding problem, or liver or kidney problems.
- If you are taking NSAIDs regularly, blood tests will be done from time to time to check your blood count (in case you are losing blood slowly from an ulcer that you may not

know about), your creatinine (for kidney function), and liver enzymes. People taking diuretics ("water pills") or ACE (angiotensin converting enzyme) inhibitors—a family of drugs that lowers blood pressure—and people with diabetes, heart failure, or existing kidney problems are more likely to have kidney problems caused by NSAIDs. These people may need more frequent blood tests to check their kidney function.

Side Effects

See NSAIDs.

Interactions with Other Drugs

See NSAIDs.

Important Information

- Taking NSAIDs with food is a good idea and may protect you from indigestion, but it does not prevent peptic ulcers.
- To minimize your GI risks, use the lowest effective dose of an NSAID.
- One of the signs that you may be bleeding from the stomach is if you have pitch-black bowel movements. Bowel movements with altered blood, in addition to being black, are also often runny and very smelly. If this happens, contact your doctor immediately.

Common Dose Sizes

Tablet: 600 mg.

Usual Adult Doses

The usual adult dose of oxaprozin is 600 mg to 1,200 mg once a day; the maximum daily dose is 1,800 mg.

Comments

See NSAIDs.

OXYCODONE

Brand Name

Roxicodone.

OxyContin is a controlled-release (slow-release) preparation of oxycodone.

Drug Family

Oxycodone is a narcotic analgesic (painkiller).

Families of Arthritis Problems Prescribed For

Oxycodone is used for moderate to severe pain, whatever the cause. Narcotic analgesics are usually prescribed only for pain that is not controlled by acetaminophen alone or an NSAID alone. Narcotics do not affect inflammation. Oxycodone is often prescribed as a combination preparation with acetaminophen (*Percocet, Roxicet, Tylox:* see ACETAMINOPHEN + NARCOTICS) or in combination with aspirin (*Percodan, Roxiprin*).

How It Works

Narcotics decrease pain by acting through specific receptors in the brain.

Avoid

Do not take oxycodone if you are allergic to it. Real allergic reactions are rare, but a lot of people get side effects, such as nausea or feeling "spacy" from oxycodone. Avoid oxycodone if you have had an addiction problem.

Take Precautions

- Do not drink alcohol while you are taking narcotics.
- There is a risk of becoming addicted to narcotics. Take the tablets only for pain. If possible, limit the dose and how long you take them. One physician should be responsible for all your narcotic prescriptions.
- Caution is needed in people with poor liver, lung, or kidney function.

Side Effects

Side effects are common with oxycodone but are usually mild. People vary in their sensitivity to different narcotics. People who cannot take preparations that contain oxycodone, for example, may be able to tolerate another preparation containing codeine, and vice versa.

Common: Nausea, vomiting, diarrhea, constipation, poor appetite, dizziness, lightheadedness or feeling "spacy," sleepiness, and fatigue are common but not serious. Low blood pressure can occur.

Less common: An allergy with rash, hives, or asthma is less common. Confusion, feeling nervous or agitated, sleeping badly, feeling "high," addictive behavior to try and get higher doses of narcotic to feel good rather than to control pain are uncommon but do occur.

Interactions with Other Drugs

Any other sedative drug: Narcotics make people sleepy, and an overdose can make people unconscious. Combining a narcotic with another sedative drug, such as alcohol, is dangerous.

Important Information

- Don't take more than the prescribed dose.

• Don't drink alcohol while you are taking narcotic painkillers.

• Narcotics may cause drowsiness and affect your concentration for driving and other tasks.

• Oxycodone is a narcotic and can be addictive (see Comments).

• Narcotics are dangerous in overdose and must be kept away from children.

• The controlled-release oxycodone tables must be swallowed whole. If you chew or crush the tablets, you could get an overdose of oxycodone.

Common Dose Sizes

Tablet: 5 mg.

Controlled-release (slow-release) tablet: 10 mg, 20 mg, 40 mg, 80 mg.

Usual Adult Doses

The usual adult dose of oxycodone is 5 to 10 mg every six hours if needed to control pain. The controlled-release (slow-release) tablet is started at a dose of 10 mg every twelve hours and can be increased if needed.

Comments

There is some controversy about how narcotic analgesics should be used to control chronic "benign" pain, meaning chronic pain not caused by cancer. This is particularly true of the strong narcotics, such as morphine, but to a lesser extent it is also true for the combination tablets containing preparations such as codeine, hydrocodone, and oxycodone. Some physicians think that the risk of addiction and abuse is high and limit narcotic prescriptions to short periods, such as a few days, in all patients. Others are less rigid and believe that these analgesics can make life bearable for some people with chronic arthritis pain that cannot be controlled by other strategies. For example, I find them helpful to control pain at night in some people with severe osteoarthritis pain who cannot take NSAIDs because of their side effects. Most rheumatologists do not prescribe narcotics for fibromyalgia because they are not particularly helpful and because they can worsen the sleep disturbance.

Addiction to these painkillers is rarely a problem if they are used to control pain. A clue to addictive behavior is if you are trying to get bigger doses of the drug and are not using them to control pain. The risk of addiction is higher in people who themselves, or whose family members, have had an addiction problem (alcohol or drugs). I have a few rules for my patients about narcotic prescriptions.

1. Use the tablets only for pain.
2. If you don't have pain, don't take them.
3. Get all your narcotic prescriptions from one doctor and from one pharmacy.
4. Escalating the dose can be an early sign of a problem.
5. Never sell, swap, or hoard tablets.
6. If you are in the position of wanting to fool doctors or do illegal things such as forging signatures to get narcotic prescriptions, things are way out of control and you need to speak with your physician about getting help.

OXYCODONE AND ACETAMINOPHEN

(PERCOCET, ROXICET, TYLOX) (see ACETAMINOPHEN + NARCOTICS)

OXYCODONE AND ASPIRIN (*CODOXY, PERCODAN, ROXIPRIN*) (SEE OXYCODONE)

OXYCONTIN (SEE OXYCODONE)

PAMELOR (NORTRIPTYLINE; SEE ***PROFILES OF COMMON ANTIDEPRESSANT DRUGS*** UNDER AMITRIPTYLINE)

PAMIDRONATE

Brand Name

Aredia.

Drug Family

Pamidronate belongs to the family of drugs that slows the resorption of bone. It is a bisphosphonate.

Families of Arthritis Problems Prescribed For

Pamidronate is mainly used to treat Paget's disease.

How It Works

Bone is continually replaced as it is resorbed and then new bone is laid down. Pamidronate slows down the resorption of bone but does not increase bone formation.

Avoid

Do not take pamidronate if you are allergic to it.

Take Precautions

Caution is needed in people with poor kidney function.

Side Effects

Common: Pamidronate is given as an intravenous infusion and can cause inflammation of the vein that it is injected into. It can lower the concentrations of calcium, phosphate, and magnesium in your blood and can cause fever. Nausea, diarrhea, and aching bones are fairly common.

Rare: An allergic rash and a low white blood cell count are rare.

Interactions with Other Drugs

Diuretics ("water pills"): Diuretics increase the frequency of low concentrations of calcium and magnesium in your blood.

Usual Adult Doses

For Paget's disease, pamidronate is usually given as a 30 mg dose, injected slowly intravenously over four hours on three consecutive days.

Comments

Because it can be given as a tablet, alendronate (*Fosamax*) is used more often than pamidronate for Paget's disease. Extra calcium and vitamin D are usually given when bisphosphonates are used to treat Paget's disease.

PAROXETINE (*PAXIL;* SEE ***PROFILES OF COMMON ANTIDEPRESSANT DRUGS*** UNDER AMITRIPTYLINE)

PENICILLAMINE

Brand Names

Cuprimine, Depen.

Sometimes Called

D-penicillamine, "D-Pen."

Drug Family

Penicillamine is a disease-modifying antirheumatic drug (DMARD).

Families of Arthritis Problems Prescribed For

Penicillamine is most often used as a DMARD to treat rheumatoid arthritis and is occasionally used to treat scleroderma (see Comments).

How It Works

We are not sure how penicillamine works in rheumatoid arthritis. Penicillamine is a "chelating agent," which means that it binds onto some of the heavy metals such as copper and lead. In fact, it is sometimes used to treat some types of heavy-metal poisoning. But we don't think that binding to heavy metals explains its effects in RA.

Avoid

Avoid penicillamine if you are allergic to it, if you have had serious bone marrow problems, or if your kidney function is poor. Penicillamine is avoided in pregnancy.

Take Precautions

- Penicillamine can cause a skin rash. If you develop a skin rash, stop the drug and contact your doctor.
- Penicillamine has to be used cautiously in people with decreased liver or kidney function.
- Your blood count and urine will be tested regularly. These tests are usually done fairly frequently, often every two

to four weeks, after you start penicillamine. After a while they will be done once a month. The white cell count and platelet count in your blood will be checked, and if they drop significantly, penicillamine may need to be stopped. Your urine will be checked for protein and, if you start to show protein in the urine, penicillamine may need to be stopped.

- Some people who are allergic to penicillin are also allergic to penicillamine.

Side Effects

Side effects are common with penicillamine, and many people who start penicillamine have to stop within a couple of years because of side effects.

Common: Skin rash, itching, hives, a metallic taste, and protein in the urine are fairly common.

Rare: Much less common but more severe are serious allergic reactions, serious bone marrow problems with a low white cell count or low platelet count, kidney problems, liver problems, optic nerve problems, muscle problems, and fever. Although it is used to treat autoimmune problems, penicillamine can rarely cause autoimmune problems. For example, penicillamine can cause drug-induced lupus and myasthenia gravis.

Interactions with Other Drugs

Other DMARDs: The risk of side effects with other DMARDs may be increased if they are used in combination with penicillamine. Penicillamine and gold are not combined.

Antacids, iron tablets, food: These can all decrease the absorption of penicillamine.

Important Information

- Monitoring is important. Don't skip your lab checkups.
- Penicillamine works slowly, but if you have had no response after four to six months of treatment, it is time to think about another DMARD.
- It is best to take penicillamine on an empty stomach.

Common Dose Sizes

Capsule: 125 mg, 250 mg.
Tablet: 250 mg.

Usual Adult Doses

The usual adult starting dose for penicillamine is 125 mg a day. The dose is increased by 125 mg every two to four weeks, up to the usual maintenance dose, which is between 375 mg and 750 mg a day. Lower doses, in the range of 250 mg to 375 mg a day, cause fewer side effects than higher doses, and some people find them effective.

Comments

Penicillamine used to be one of the few drugs we had that were effective against RA. In the 1980s many people with RA were on penicillamine, but now penicillamine has largely been replaced by safer and more effective treatments such as methotrexate. Most rheumatologists have only a handful of patients who are still taking penicillamine. In most people penicillamine is not very effective, and side effects are common. Penicillamine works slowly in RA, and it may be six to twelve weeks before you see a response. It is debated whether penicillamine is useful for scleroderma. My interpretation of the evidence is that it is probably not effective, but some rheumatologists believe that it helps to reduce skin tightness.

PERCOCET (SEE ACETAMINOPHEN + NARCOTICS)

PERCODAN (SEE OXYCODONE)

PHENYLBUTAZONE

Brand Names

Butazolidin, Butazone.

Drug Family

Phenylbutazone is a nonsteroidal anti-inflammatory drug (NSAID). There are two big groups of NSAIDs, divided by whether they inhibit both cyclo-oxygenase (COX) enzymes, COX-1 and COX-2, or are more selective for COX-2. Phenylbutazone inhibits both COX-1 and COX-2.

Families of Arthritis Problems Prescribed For

NSAIDs are used to treat all kinds of pain and inflammation, whether they affect the joints or not, but phenylbutazone, because of its side effects, is used only for the very occasional person who has ankylosing spondylitis that is not responding to other NSAIDs. Phenylbutazone has a reputation for sometimes helping people with ankylosing spondylitis whose pain is not controlled by other NSAIDs. Phenylbutazone, like other NSAIDs, decreases pain and inflammation but does not change the progression of arthritis.

How It Works

Most NSAIDs inhibit the enzymes COX-1 and COX-2. Inhibiting these cyclo-oxygenase enzymes decreases the formation of chemicals called prostaglandins. Decreasing the prostaglandins made by COX-2 is anti-inflammatory, which is usually why we use NSAIDs. Inhibiting COX-1 makes platelets in your blood less sticky, which is why aspirin is used to treat heart attacks. COX-1 also protects the stomach from ulcers, and blocking COX-1 may be why the risk of peptic ulcers is increased with many NSAIDs.

Avoid

Do not take phenylbutazone if you are allergic to it or if you have had bone-marrow problems. People who have had a serious allergic reaction (swelling of the face and tongue, and wheezing) to one NSAID can have the same reaction to others. People with asthma or nasal polyps are more likely to be allergic to NSAIDs. NSAIDs are avoided if someone has an active peptic ulcer, is bleeding, or is pregnant.

Take Precautions

- NSAIDs can cause fluid retention and can worsen heart failure and high blood pressure.
- Some people are at higher risk for peptic ulcers caused by NSAIDs. Risk factors are being older than 65 years, having had a previous peptic ulcer, having had a previous bleeding ulcer, and taking a corticosteroid. In people at higher risk for peptic ulcers caused by NSAIDs, most rheumatologists would avoid an NSAID, if possible. If this is not possible, then prescribing misoprostol (see MISOPROSTOL—*Cytotec*) or a proton pump inhibitor (see OMEPRAZOLE—*Prilosec*) to protect against peptic ulcers caused by NSAIDs is an option. Another option is to use a COX-2 selective NSAID (see CELECOXIB—*Celebrex* and ROFECOXIB—*Vioxx*). None of these choices is foolproof, and peptic ulcers can still happen.

• NSAIDs have to be used carefully in people who have asthma, a bleeding problem, or liver or kidney problems.

• If you are taking NSAIDs regularly, blood tests will be done from time to time to check your blood count (in case you are losing blood slowly from an ulcer that you may not know about), your creatinine (for kidney function), and liver enzymes. People taking diuretics ("water pills") or ACE (angiotensin converting enzyme) inhibitors—a family of drugs that lowers blood pressure—and people with diabetes, heart failure, or existing kidney problems are more likely to have kidney problems caused by NSAIDs. These people may need more frequent blood tests to check their kidney function.

Side Effects

See NSAIDs.

Phenylbutazone can rarely cause serious problems with the bone marrow so that it does not make red blood cells, white blood cells, and platelets.

Interactions with Other Drugs

See NSAIDs.

Important Information

• Taking NSAIDs with food is a good idea and may protect you from indigestion, but it does not prevent peptic ulcers.

• To minimize your gastrointestinal (GI) risks, use the lowest effective dose of an NSAID.

• One of the signs that you may be bleeding from the stomach is if you have pitch-black bowel movements. Bowel movements with altered blood, in addition to being black, are also often runny and very smelly. If this happens, contact your doctor immediately.

• Bone marrow damage from phenylbutazone is rare, but when it occurs it can be very sudden and can happen even if your blood count has been checked regularly. If you are taking phenylbutazone and develop severe mouth sores, infection, bleeding, or feel faint, contact your physician immediately.

Common D e Sizes

Tablet: 100 mg.

Usual Adult Doses

The usual adult dose of phenylbutazone is 100 mg three or four times a day.

Comments

Phenylbutazone, because of the serious bone marrow problems that it can cause, and because alternative NSAIDs are available, is very seldom prescribed. We do not understand why phenylbutazone may help some people with ankylosing spondylitis who have not responded to other NSAIDs. Phenylbutazone should be prescribed only by rheumatologists. Even then, it should be prescribed for only selected people, after the risks and benefits have been discussed and after other NSAIDs have failed.

PILOCARPINE

Brand Name

Salagen.

Sometimes Called

Pilocarpine hydrochloride.

Drug Family

Pilocarpine stimulates nerves to certain parts of your body, particularly the glands that make saliva.

Families of Arthritis Problems Prescribed For

Pilocarpine is used to treat the dry mouth that is often a problem for people with Sjogren's syndrome.

How It Works

Pilocarpine stimulates the cholinergic nerves to the glands that make your saliva so that they make more saliva.

Avoid

Do not take pilocarpine if you are allergic to it. Pilocarpine is avoided in people who have a certain type of glaucoma (increased pressure in the eyeball) called "narrow-angle glaucoma."

Take Precautions

- Caution is needed in people who have heart problems, asthma, chronic bronchitis, and other types of lung problems.
- Caution is needed in people who have gallstones or kidney stones.

Side Effects

Pilocarpine often causes side effects. These are usually nuisance side effects that are not serious, but they do stop some people from taking it.

Common: The most common side effect of pilocarpine is sweating. This is because it also stimulates the nerves to the sweat glands. Pilocarpine can cause dizziness, headache, blurred vision, gastrointestinal problems such as nausea or diarrhea, passing urine more often, feeling flushed, and a runny nose or blocked nose.

Interactions with Other Drugs

Ipratrobium *(Atrovent):* Pilocarpine can antagonize the effects of ipratrobium, an inhaled drug used to treat asthma.

Important Information

- If you sweat excessively while you are taking pilocarpine, make sure that you keep up your fluid intake.

Common Dose Sizes

Tablet: 5 mg.

Usual Adult Doses

The usual adult dose of pilocarpine is one 5 mg tablet taken three or four times a day.

Comments

About half the people with Sjogren's syndrome notice a significant improvement in their symptoms with pilocarpine. The symptom of dry mouth improves most often, but sometimes other problems such as dry eyes and dry skin also improve. Pilocarpine treats symptoms; it does not affect the underlying cause of the symptoms.

PIROXICAM

Brand Name

Feldene.

Drug Family

Piroxicam is a nonsteroidal anti-inflammatory drug (NSAID). There are two big groups of NSAIDs, divided by whether they inhibit both cyclo-oxygenase (COX) enzymes, COX-1 and COX-2, or are more selective for COX-2. Piroxicam inhibits both COX-1 and COX-2.

Families of Arthritis Problems Prescribed For

NSAIDs are used to treat all kinds of pain and inflammation, whether they affect the joints or not. NSAIDs are used to treat many kinds of arthritis problems, such as RA, gout, ankylosing spondylitis, osteoarthritis, and bursitis. NSAIDs decrease pain and inflammation, but they do not change the progression of arthritis.

How It Works

Most NSAIDs inhibit the enzymes COX-1 and COX-2. Inhibiting these cyclo-oxygenase enzymes decreases the formation of chemicals called prostaglandins. Decreasing the prostaglandins made by COX-2 is anti-inflammatory, which is usually why we use NSAIDs. Inhibiting COX-1 makes platelets in your blood less sticky, which is why aspirin is used to treat heart attacks. COX-1 also protects the stomach from ulcers, and blocking COX-1 may be why the risk of peptic ulcers is increased with many NSAIDs.

Avoid

Do not take piroxicam if you are allergic to it. People who have had a serious allergic reaction (swelling of the face and tongue, and wheezing) to one NSAID can have the same reaction with others. People with asthma or nasal polyps are more likely to be allergic to NSAIDs. NSAIDs are avoided if someone has an active peptic ulcer, is bleeding, or is pregnant.

Take Precautions

• NSAIDs can cause fluid retention and can worsen heart failure and high blood pressure.

• Some people are at higher risk for peptic ulcers caused by NSAIDs. Risk factors are being older than 65 years, having had a previous peptic ulcer, having had a previous bleeding ulcer, and taking a corticosteroid. In people at higher risk for peptic ulcers caused by NSAIDs, most rheumatologists would avoid an NSAID, if possible. If this is not possible, then prescribing misoprostol (see MISOPROSTOL—*Cytotec*) or a proton pump inhibitor (see OMEPRAZOLE—*Prilosec*) to protect against peptic ulcers caused by NSAIDs is an option. Another option is to use a COX-2 selective NSAID (see CELECOXIB—*Celebrex* and ROFECOXIB—*Vioxx*). None of these choices is foolproof, and peptic ulcers can still happen.

• NSAIDs have to be used carefully in people who have asthma, a bleeding problem, or liver or kidney problems.

• If you are taking NSAIDs regularly, blood tests will be done from time to time to check your blood count (in case you are losing blood slowly from an ulcer that you may not know about), your creatinine (for kidney function), and liver enzymes. People taking diuretics ("water pills") or ACE (angiotensin converting enzyme) inhibitors—a family of drugs that lowers blood pressure—and people with diabetes, heart failure, or existing kidney problems are more likely to have kidney problems caused by NSAIDs. These people may need more frequent blood tests to check their kidney function.

Side Effects

See NSAIDs.

Interactions with Other Drugs

See NSAIDs.

Important Information

• Taking NSAIDs with food is a good idea and may protect you from indigestion, but it does not prevent peptic ulcers.

• To minimize your GI risks, use the lowest effective dose of an NSAID.

• One of the signs that you may be bleeding from the stomach is if you have pitch-black bowel movements. Bowel movements with altered blood, in addition to being black, are also often runny and very smelly. If this happens, contact your doctor immediately.

Common Dose Sizes

Capsule: 10 mg, 20 mg.

Usual Adult Doses

The usual adult dose of piroxicam is 10 to 20 mg taken once a day or split into two doses.

Comments

See NSAIDs.

PLAQUENIL (SEE HYDROXYCHLOROQUINE)

PREDNISOLONE (SEE CORTICOSTEROIDS)

PREDNISONE (SEE CORTICOSTEROIDS)

PROBENECID

Brand Names

Benemid, Probalan.

Drug Family

Probenecid belongs to the family of drugs that lowers uric acid levels in your body.

Families of Arthritis Problems Prescribed For

Probenecid is used to decrease the uric acid levels in your body, and by doing this it prevents attacks of gout.

How It Works

Probenecid is called a uricosuric drug because it gets rid of uric acid from your body by increasing the uric acid concentration in the urine.

Avoid

Do not take probenecid if you are allergic to it or have poor kidney function.

Take Precautions

- Caution is needed in people with active peptic ulcers.
- A blood test is usually taken from time to time to check your uric acid level. The drop in the uric acid level after treatment can be a useful guide to how effective the treatment is.

Side Effects

Common: Gastrointestinal symptoms such as nausea are common. Vomiting and headache are less common.

Rare: A rash, itching, an allergic reaction, bringing on an attack of gout, bone marrow problems, and kidney problems are rare.

Interactions with Other Drugs

Aspirin and other salicylates: These drugs can block the way probenecid helps your body get rid of uric acid.

Penicillin and cephalosporin antibiotics: Probenecid

increases the blood levels of these antibiotics. This is not usually a problem except in people who have poor kidney function.

Methotrexate: Probenecid increases the levels of methotrexate and increases the risk of side effects from methotrexate.

Acyclovir *(Zovirax)* and other antiviral drugs: Probenecid can increase the levels of these drugs.

Important Information

- Probenecid is taken regularly to prevent gout. Your risk for getting gout does not usually go away. So to keep attacks of gout away, probenecid often needs to be taken for many years, or indefinitely. Probenecid may not completely prevent attacks of acute gout. If you have an attack of gout while you are taking probenecid, remember that probenecid has no effect on the pain and swelling of the acute attack. A common mistake people make is to take their probenecid only when they get an attack of gout.
- Drink plenty of fluids. Probenecid increases the uric acid concentrations in your urine, and keeping your urine dilute will decrease your risk of getting uric acid kidney stones.

Common Dose Sizes

Tablet: 500 mg.

Usual Adult Doses

The usual adult starting dose of probenecid is 250 mg twice a day, and the dose is increased slowly, if needed, usually to somewhere between 500 mg and 1 g twice a day.

Comments

Drugs that decrease the concentration of uric acid in your body, such as probenecid, *prevent* attacks of gout. These drugs do nothing for the acute pain of gout. They are trying to fix the problem. This means you have to take them regularly, no matter how your gout is doing. Not everyone who has an attack of gout is treated with drugs to lower their uric acid. Some people have only one attack of gout in their lifetime. If someone has two or more attacks in a year or two, most rheumatologists would start preventive treatment. Colchicine or a nonsteroidal anti-inflammatory drug is also usually prescribed for the first three to twelve months of probenecid treatment because there is a higher risk of an acute attack of gout coming on when treatment to lower the uric acid level is started. In people with gout who have tophi or uric acid kidney stones, allopurinol is preferred to probenecid.

PROPOXYPHENE

Brand Names

Darvon and many others.

Drug Family

Propoxyphene is a narcotic analgesic (painkiller). It is often prescribed in combination with acetaminophen (see ACETAMINOPHEN + NARCOTICS).

PROPULSID (SEE CISAPRIDE)

PROSORBA COLUMN

Brand Name

Prosorba Column.

Sometimes Called

Protein A Immunoadsorption Column.

Drug Family

The *Prosorba* column is one of the more recently approved treatments for RA. It seems to act like a disease-modifying antirheumatic drug (DMARD). It is not a drug, in the sense that it is not something that you swallow or inject. Your blood is drawn out of a vein in your arm, passed through the column, and re-injected.

Families of Arthritis Problems Prescribed For

The *Prosorba* column is used to treat RA in people who do not respond to or are unable to take DMARDs. It is also used to treat people with a very low platelet count that is caused by antibodies to their platelets—a condition called idiopathic thrombocytopenic purpura, or ITP.

How It Works

Your blood is passed through the *Prosorba* column to remove certain proteins that promote RA. These proteins stick onto proteins in the column, so when your blood is injected back into your body, it has been "purified." The column contains a protein, called protein A, from a common type of bacterium, staphylococcus. The column works a bit like a filter, but we are not sure exactly which proteins are being removed.

Avoid

You should avoid *Prosorba* column treatment if you

- have had allergic problems with apheresis (the procedure of having your blood drawn out, having something done to it, and then injected back into you).
- are on angiotensin converting enzyme (ACE) inhibitors (a family of drugs that lowers blood pressure).
- have problems with forming blood clots too easily (hypercoagulability).

Take Precautions

• Caution is needed in people with heart, kidney, or blood pressure problems in which changes in blood pressure or the amount of fluid in your body could be harmful.

• Caution is needed in people who have low blood pressure, are anemic, or have an active infection.

Side Effects

Common: Access to veins can be a problem in some people. You need to have good veins so that IV lines can be put in to take out some of your blood and then later pump it back in. People who do not have good veins in their arms sometimes need what is called a central line. A central line is an IV tube that is put into one of the big veins in the neck or under the collar bone and can be left in place for weeks or sometimes months.

Many of these central lines have become infected or caused clotting problems in people with RA who got apheresis. If possible, central lines should be avoided in people who are going to be treated with the *Prosorba* column.

The apheresis itself, with or without the *Prosorba* column, often causes minor side effects such as joint pain, fatigue, nausea, rash, low blood pressure, feeling flushed, dizziness, tingling, fever, and chills. Most people can tolerate these side effects, which do not last long.

Interactions with Other Drugs

ACE inhibitors: If you are taking an ACE inhibitor or have recently taken one, you should not have *Prosorba* column treatment. Potentially fatal problems such as low blood pressure and shock can occur if someone on an ACE inhibitor has apheresis. The manufacturer recommends a minimum period of seventy-two hours between stopping an ACE inhibitor and starting *Prosorba* column treatment, but a longer "washout" may be safer.

DMARDs: We do not know how the *Prosorba* column affects the response to DMARDs.

Important Information

- An arthritis flare immediately after a treatment is common but usually settles quickly.
- Most of the side effects occur during the actual apheresis treatment and are caused by the process of drawing off your blood and then giving it back to you.
- The response to *Prosorba* treatment in RA is slow, taking eight to twelve weeks, but can be prolonged, sometimes lasting twenty weeks or longer after the treatments have been stopped.

Usual Adult Doses

Prosorba column treatment is usually given once a week for twelve weeks.

Comments

There are many unanswered questions about this treatment. We do not know exactly how it works, but that is also true for many RA treatments. Relatively few people with RA have been treated with the *Prosorba* column, so there is not a lot of information about either response or safety or what happens when people are retreated after the effect of one course of treatment has worn off. How effective is this treatment? I don't know. Very few people have been studied. The published results are not very impressive, with 32 percent of people improving their overall arthritis score by at least 20 percent, compared with about 10 percent of people who got apheresis without the *Prosorba* column. However, these numbers may underestimate what happens in the clinic because the people studied had very severe RA that had not responded to other treatments. Limited information, expense, and the inconvenience of setting up the apheresis treatment are reasons why relatively few people with RA are treated with the *Prosorba* column.

PROTON PUMP INHIBITORS (SEE OMEPRAZOLE)

PROZAC (FLUOXETINE; SEE *PROFILES OF COMMON ANTIDEPRESSANT DRUGS* UNDER AMITRIPTYLINE)

RABEPRAZOLE (*ACIPHEX;* SEE *PROFILES OF COMMON PROTON PUMP INHIBITORS* UNDER OMEPRAZOLE)

RALOXIFENE

Brand Name

Evista.

Drug Family

Raloxifene is a selective estrogen receptor modulator (SERM), one of a new class of drug that acts on the estrogen receptors in bone but does not stimulate the estrogen receptors in the breasts or uterus.

Families of Arthritis Problems Prescribed For

Raloxifene is used to treat and prevent osteoporosis in women who have gone through the menopause. Remember that osteoporosis means "thin bones" and is not a type of arthritis. The aim of treating osteoporosis is to prevent fractures. Raloxifene is used particularly in women who would otherwise take estrogen replacement treatment but who cannot or do not want to take estrogens.

How It Works

SERMs stimulate some of the estrogen receptors in your body, particularly the receptors in bone, without stimulating estrogen receptors in other places, such as the breasts or uterus.

Avoid

Do not take raloxifene if you are allergic to it. Raloxifene is avoided in pregnancy. People who have had problems with blood clots, such as a blood clot in the leg (deep vein thrombosis), in the lung (pulmonary embolus), or in the eye (retinal vein thrombosis), should not take raloxifene.

Take Precautions

- If you know you are going to be sitting or lying still for a long time, for example if you are going to have surgery, stop the raloxifene at least three days before this, and restart it only when you are active and on your feet again.

Side Effects

Common: Hot flashes and leg cramps.

Rare: Blood clots, such as blood clots in the veins (deep vein thrombosis).

Interactions with Other Drugs

Estrogens: Combining estrogen hormone replacement with a SERM, such as raloxifene, is avoided.

Cholestyramine (*Questran*): If cholestyramine and raloxifene are used together, the raloxifene is not absorbed well.

Important Information

- Raloxifene slightly increases the risk of you getting a blood clot. If you get a painful swollen calf or suddenly get chest pain or become very short of breath, contact your doctor immediately.
- Raloxifene does not decrease symptoms of menopause such as hot flashes. In some people it can bring them on.

Common Dose Sizes

Tablet: 60 mg.

Usual Adult Doses

The usual adult dose of raloxifene is one 60 mg tablet taken every day.

Comments

Osteoporosis is a common problem, particularly in women after the menopause, and in people who are taking corticosteroids. Osteoporosis is diagnosed by measuring your bone density, often with a type of scan known as a DEXA. The usual program to treat or prevent osteoporosis also includes stopping smoking and alcohol, increasing exercise, and taking calcium supplements and a low dose of vitamin D, often as part of a multivitamin tablet.

Raloxifene does increase bone density and decreases your risk of fractures, but there is stronger evidence showing that estrogens and alendronate decrease the risk of fractures. Don't forget that the aim of treating osteoporosis is to prevent fractures and that many fractures are caused by falls. Simple things can reduce your risk of falling. Some of these may apply to you. Get rid of loose throw rugs and other objects that can trip you, have nonslip surfaces, use a cane if you need one, don't hurry—that telephone can keep ringing—and keep a night-light on so that you can see your way to the bathroom. People with poor vision are more likely to fall, so have your vision checked from time to time. Alcohol and medicines that affect your balance, such as many kinds of sleeping pills, increase your risk of falling. Avoid them if possible.

Raloxifene, like estrogens, can improve your cholesterol profile a little. Some experts argue that the improvement in the cholesterol profile is greater with estrogens than it is with raloxifene; others disagree. A big advantage of raloxifene over estrogens is that raloxifene does not stimulate estrogen receptors in the breasts or uterus; in fact, raloxifene blocks estrogen receptors in the breasts. So there is no vaginal bleeding and no increased risk of breast cancer; rather, the evidence suggests that raloxifene lowers the risk of breast cancer. There are clinical trials running to see if raloxifene can be used to prevent breast cancer.

RANITIDINE (*ZANTAC;* SEE ***PROFILES OF COMMON H_2-RECEPTOR ANTAGONIST DRUGS*** UNDER CIMETIDINE)

REFRESH (SEE ARTIFICIAL TEARS)

RELAFEN (SEE NABUMETONE)

REMICADE (SEE INFLIXIMAB)

RHEUMATREX (SEE METHOTREXATE)

RIDAURA (SEE AURANOFIN)

RISEDRONATE

Brand Name
Actonel

Drug Family
Risedronate belongs to the family of drugs that prevent bone loss. It is a bisphosphonate.

Families of Arthritis Problems Prescribed For
Risedronate is used to treat and prevent osteoporosis. Remember that osteoporosis means thin bones and is not a type of arthritis. The aim of treating osteoporosis is to prevent fractures. Risedronate is also used to treat Paget's disease.

How it works
Bone is continually replaced as it is absorbed, and then new bone is laid down to replace it. Risedronate slows down the resorption of bone but does not increase bone formation. Risedronate stabilizes bone density or increases it slightly. In clinical trials risedronate cuts the risk of fractures caused by osteoporosis by about half.

Avoid
Do not take risedronate if you are allergic to it, have poor kidney function, or have a low blood calcium level.

Take Precautions
Risedronate does not seem to cause serious gastrointestinal problems very often but caution is advised if you have a hiatal hernia or acid reflux (sometimes called GERD or gastroesophageal reflux disease). Risedronate needs to be taken exactly as directed otherwise it will not get into your blood-

stream and will not work, or it may reflux up your esophagus (the food pipe that joins your mouth to your stomach) and cause irritation there.

Side Effects

Common: Mild stomach (GI) upset such as nausea, diarrhea, gas, constipation and indigestion are common. You may notice some aching in your muscles, back or joints or feel as if you have the flu

Rare: An allergic rash or low blood calcium level are rare.

Interactions with Other Drugs

NSAIDs: GI side effects may be more common when risedronate and NSAIDs are used together. However, many people with both rheumatoid arthritis and osteoporosis have taken risedronate and an NSAID and tolerated the combination well.

Any drug: Risedronate is not absorbed into your body if you take it at the same time as any other drug or with food.

Important Information

- Risedronate should be taken with a full glass of water first thing in the morning.
- Do not eat or drink anything other than water for at least 30 minutes after taking risedronate. Even coffee or fruit juice stop the risedronate from getting into your body. If you can wait an hour before eating or drinking something else, so much the better, because more risedronate will be absorbed into your body.
- After you have taken risedronate, stay upright and don't go back to bed. This is so that the tablet doesn't reflux back up your esophagus.
- Take risedronate by itself, not with your other medicines. Delay taking your other medicines for at least an hour.

Common Dose Sizes

Tablet: 30 mg (to treat Paget's disease) and 5 mg (to treat and prevent osteoporosis).

Usual Adult Doses

The usual adult dose of risedronate for osteoporosis is 5 mg a day.

The usual dose of risedronate for Paget's disease is 30 mg a day for 2 months. This often controls Paget's disease, but if it relapses, another course of treatment may be needed.

Comments

Osteoporosis is a common problem, particularly in women after the menopause and in people taking corticosteroids. Osteoporosis is diagnosed by measuring your bone density, often with a type of scan known as a DEXA (dual-energy X-ray absorptiometry). The usual program to treat or prevent osteoporosis also includes stopping smoking and alcohol, increasing exercise, and taking calcium supplements and a low dose of vitamin D, often as part of a multivitamin tablet.

Alendronate is the bisphosphonate that has the most supporting evidence showing that it decreases the risk of fractures but in clinical trials risedronate seems equally effective. Don't forget that the aim of treating osteoporosis is to prevent fractures and that many fractures are caused by falls. Simple things can reduce your risk of falling. Some of these may apply to you. Get rid of loose throw rugs and other objects that can trip you, have nonslip surfaces, use a cane if you need one, don't hurry—that telephone can keep ringing—and keep a night-light on so that you can see your way to the bathroom. People with poor vision are more likely to fall, so have your vision checked from time to time. Alcohol and medicines that affect your balance, such as many kinds of sleeping pills, increase your risk of falling. Avoid them if possible.

Risedronate seems to cause GI side effects less often than alendronate but so far there is not much experience with the drug outside of clinical trials. If risedronate does cause less GI problems than alendronate and is equally effective this will be an advantage.

ROBAXIN (SEE METHOCARBAMOL)

ROFECOXIB

Brand Name

Vioxx.

Drug Family

Rofecoxib belongs to the nonsteroidal anti-inflammatory drug (NSAID) family. There are two big groups of NSAIDs, divided by whether they inhibit both cyclo-oxygenase (COX) enzymes, COX-1 and COX-2, or are more selective for COX-2. Rofecoxib is selective for COX-2 and has little effect on COX-1.

Families of Arthritis Problems Prescribed For

NSAIDs are used to treat all kinds of pain and inflammation, whether they affect the joints or not. NSAIDs are used to treat many kinds of arthritis problems, such as RA, osteoarthritis, and bursitis. NSAIDs decrease pain and inflammation, but they do not change the progression of arthritis.

How It Works

Most NSAIDs inhibit the enzymes COX-1 and COX-2, but selective NSAIDs, such as rofecoxib, are more selective for COX-2. Inhibiting these cyclo-oxygenase enzymes decreases the formation of chemicals called prostaglandins. Decreasing the prostaglandins made by COX-2 is anti-inflammatory, which is usually why we use NSAIDs. NSAIDs that inhibit COX-1 make platelets in your blood less sticky, which is why aspirin is used to treat heart attacks. COX-1 also protects the stomach from ulcers, so blocking COX-1 may be why the nonselective NSAIDs increase the risk of peptic ulcers. Because rofecoxib selectively blocks COX-2, it is kinder on the stomach than nonselective NSAIDs and also does not make platelets less sticky.

Avoid

Do not take rofecoxib if you are allergic to it. People who have had a serious allergic reaction (swelling of the face and tongue, and wheezing) to one NSAID can have the same reaction to other NSAIDs. People with asthma or nasal polyps are more likely to be allergic to NSAIDs. NSAIDs are avoided if someone has an active peptic ulcer or is pregnant.

Take Precautions

- NSAIDs can cause fluid retention and can worsen heart failure and high blood pressure.
- Some people are at higher risk for peptic ulcers caused by NSAIDs. Risk factors are being older than 65 years, having had a previous peptic ulcer, having had a previous bleeding ulcer, and taking a corticosteroid. In people who have a higher risk for peptic ulcers caused by NSAIDs, most rheumatologists would avoid NSAIDs if possible. If this is not possible, then prescribing misoprostol (see MISOPROSTOL— *Cytotec*) or a proton pump inhibitor (see OMEPRAZOLE—*Prilosec*) to protect against peptic ulcers caused by NSAIDs is an option. Another option is to use a COX-2 selective NSAID such as ROFECOXIB *(Vioxx)* or CELECOXIB (*Celebrex*). None of these choices is foolproof, and peptic ulcers can still happen.

• NSAIDs, even COX-2 selective NSAIDs, have to be used carefully in people who have asthma or liver or kidney problems.

• If you are taking NSAIDs regularly, blood tests will be done from time to time to check your blood count (in case you are losing blood slowly from an ulcer that you may not know about), your creatinine (for kidney function), and liver enzymes. People taking diuretics ("water pills") or ACE (angiotensin converting enzyme) inhibitors—a family of drugs that lowers blood pressure—and people with diabetes, heart failure, or existing kidney problems are more likely to have kidney problems caused by NSAIDs. These people may need more frequent blood tests to check their kidney function.

Side Effects

Common: NSAIDs are one of the most common medicines we take. Many people tolerate NSAIDs reasonably well. Gastrointestinal problems, usually indigestion or heartburn pain, are the most common reasons people stop NSAIDs. One of the less common but more severe side effects is a serious peptic ulcer problem. When GI problems are measured by symptoms such as indigestion or by the number of small ulcers seen on endoscopy, rofecoxib, one of the selective COX-2 blocking NSAIDs, clearly causes fewer GI problems than nonselective NSAIDs. The risk of serious bleeding from peptic ulcers is probably also lower with selective COX-2 blocking NSAIDs such as rofecoxib than it is with nonselective NSAIDs. NSAIDs often cause some fluid retention with a little ankle swelling.

Less common: Peptic ulcers can be silent, without warning symptoms such as indigestion. Small ulcers occur in many people taking NSAIDs without their even knowing it. In people at higher risk (older than 65 years, a previous peptic ulcer, a previous bleeding ulcer, and combined treatment with a corticosteroid), the annual risk of a serious ulcer problem with nonselective NSAIDs can be as high as three out of every 100 people. It is not yet clear how these numbers apply to selective COX-2 blocking NSAIDs such as rofecoxib, but it is likely that the risk will be lower.

Blood pressure can increase in some people, usually by a small amount. Abnormal liver function tests (usually mild), rashes, ringing in the ears, and a feeling of lightheadedness or feeling "spacy" can occur.

Rare: Bleeding from an ulcer, perforation of the bowel, serious liver problems, rash, dizziness, and kidney problems can occur. People who have an allergic reaction to one NSAID and get wheezing, a lumpy and itchy rash, and swelling of the tongue or face are often allergic to other NSAIDs.

Interactions with Other Drugs

Warfarin *(Coumadin):* Rofecoxib, unlike the nonselective NSAIDs, does not make platelets less sticky. But because there is still a small risk of peptic ulcers that can bleed, rofecoxib is avoided, if possible, in people taking warfarin or other anticoagulants. Rofecoxib slightly increases the anticoagulant (anti-blood clotting) effect of warfarin in some people. If you are taking warfarin to prevent blood clots and start taking rofecoxib, you may need to have your blood monitored more frequently than usual, and your dose of warfarin may need to be changed.

NSAIDs: A combination of two NSAIDs is avoided because it does not improve the control of inflammation but does increase the risk of side effects. Rofecoxib has no effects on platelets, so if someone needs aspirin to prevent a heart attack or stroke, a low dose of aspirin is often prescribed with rofecoxib.

Lithium: Many NSAIDs can increase lithium levels. Lithium levels are usually monitored, and the dose of lithium can be decreased if needed.

Diuretics ("water pills") or ACE (angiotensin converting enzyme) inhibitors—a family of drugs that lowers blood pressure: Many NSAIDs blunt the ability of these drugs to lower blood pressure.

Methotrexate: Rofecoxib, in a dose higher than is usually used, increased the blood levels of methotrexate by about 25 percent. In rheumatology practice, with the low doses of methotrexate used, this interaction may not be important in most people.

Rifampin *(Rifadin, Rimactane):* Rifampin increases the speed at which your liver breaks down rofecoxib, and you may need larger doses.

Important Information

- The risks of peptic ulcers from NSAIDs are much lower with selective COX-2 inhibitors than they are with nonselective NSAIDs, but remember that they can still happen.
- Taking NSAIDs with food is a good idea and may protect you from indigestion, but it does not prevent peptic ulcers.
- To minimize your gastrointestinal risks, use the lowest effective dose of an NSAID.
- One of the signs that you may be bleeding from the stomach is if you have pitch-black bowel movements. Bowel movements with altered blood, in addition to being black, are also often runny and very smelly. If this happens, contact your doctor immediately.

Common Dose Sizes

Tablet: 12.5 mg, 25 mg.

Usual Adult Doses

The usual adult dose of rofecoxib is 12.5 mg once a day. The maximum recommended dose is 25 mg a day.

Comments

Most people take NSAIDs for arthritis pain. There is no convincing evidence that one NSAID is more effective than another for arthritis pain. COX-2 selective NSAIDs, such as rofecoxib, are about as effective as others. There is no evidence that they are more effective. But people respond differently, and you may find that one particular NSAID suits you much better than any of the others. People who are allergic to sulfonamides ("sulfa drugs") can take rofecoxib, but they may be allergic to celecoxib. There are many NSAIDs on the market. I don't think there is much point in trying a lot of different NSAIDs to get greater effect. If two or three NSAIDs don't help much, it usually means that some other type of treatment may be better for you.

Some people with osteoarthritis find that NSAIDs and acetaminophen reduce their pain by about the same amount. If this is the case for you, take acetaminophen because it is safer. Rheumatoid arthritis causes a lot more inflammation than osteoarthritis, and NSAIDs usually control the symptoms of RA better than acetaminophen does. People vary a lot. Some people with RA tell me they find that NSAIDs make very little difference to their symptom control. For them the risks outweigh the benefits, and I suggest that they need not take an NSAID. Other people with RA find that NSAIDs help them a lot, and for them NSAIDs are very useful. RA is virtually never controlled by an NSAID alone, so a DMARD is introduced early in the treatment plan.

There are many unanswered questions about NSAIDs. Do the serious ulcer problems caused by older, nonselective NSAIDs in relatively few people mean that everyone should be treated with a new COX-2 selective NSAID, although it may cost more? Are there side effects from the new COX-2 inhibitor NSAIDs that we don't know about yet? In people at higher risk for peptic ulcers, are COX-2 selective NSAIDs safer than a nonselective NSAID taken with a stomach protective agent such as misoprostol? We don't know the answers to these questions. My approach is not to change people who are stable on their older NSAID to a newer COX-2 selective drug. In people at higher risk for NSAID ulcer problems, I discuss the choices available and either use a COX-2 selective drug or an older NSAID with either misoprostol (see MISOPROSTOL—*Cytotec*) or a proton pump inhibitor (see OMEPRAZOLE—*Prilosec*) to protect against ulcers. As more information becomes available, we will have clearer answers to these questions. I suspect that COX-2 selective NSAIDs, because they are equally effective and are likely to be safer, will replace nonselective NSAIDs as the first choice for most people with arthritis who need NSAIDs.

SALAGEN (SEE PILOCARPINE)

SALSALATE

Brand Names

Argesic-SA, Disalcid, Salflex.

Drug Family

Salsalate belongs to the NSAID subfamily called nonacetylated salicylates, which behaves a little differently from other NSAIDs.

Families of Arthritis Problems Prescribed For

Nonacetylated salicylates are used as NSAIDs to treat rheumatoid arthritis and osteoarthritis. Nonacetylated salicylates are chemically very similar to aspirin but have slight differences in their structure that change the way they work and their side effects.

How It Works

It is not clear how nonacetylated salicylates work. Unlike other NSAIDs, they are only weak inhibitors of the cyclooxygenase (COX) enzymes that make prostaglandins. They probably have some of their effect by either blocking or slowing the formation of COX-2.

Avoid

Do not take nonacetylated salicylates if you are allergic to aspirin or other salicylates. People who have had a serious allergic reaction (swelling of the face and tongue, and wheezing) to one NSAID can have the same reaction to others. People with asthma or nasal polyps are more likely to be allergic to NSAIDs. Salicylates are avoided in children and if someone has an active peptic ulcer, is bleeding, or is pregnant.

Take Precautions

- NSAIDs can cause fluid retention and can worsen heart failure and high blood pressure.
- Some people are at higher risk for peptic ulcers caused by NSAIDs. Risk factors are being older than 65 years, having had a previous peptic ulcer, having had a previous bleeding ulcer, and taking a corticosteroid. In people at higher risk for peptic ulcers caused by NSAIDs, most rheumatologists would avoid an NSAID, if possible. If this is not possible, then prescribing misoprostol (see MISOPROSTOL—*Cytotec*) or a proton pump inhibitor (see OMEPRAZOLE—*Prilosec*) to protect against peptic ulcers caused by NSAIDs is an option. Another option is to use a COX-2 selective NSAID (see CELECOXIB—*Celebrex*

and ROFECOXIB—*Vioxx*). None of these choices is foolproof, and peptic ulcers can still happen.

• Salicylates have to be used carefully in people who have asthma, a bleeding problem, or liver or kidney problems.

• If you are taking NSAIDs regularly, blood tests will be done from time to time to check your blood count (in case you are losing blood slowly from an ulcer that you may not know about), your creatinine (for kidney function), and liver enzymes. People taking diuretics ("water pills") or ACE (angiotensin converting enzyme) inhibitors—a family of drugs that lowers blood pressure—and people with diabetes, heart failure, or existing kidney problems are more likely to have kidney problems caused by NSAIDs. These people may need more frequent blood tests to check their kidney function.

Side Effects

Common: Stomach irritation causing indigestion, heartburn, and stomach pain is common. NSAIDs often cause some fluid retention with a little ankle swelling.

Less common: Peptic ulcers can be silent, without warning symptoms such as indigestion. In people at higher risk (older than 65 years, a previous peptic ulcer, a previous bleeding ulcer, and taking a corticosteroid), the risk of an ulcer problem with aspirin and other nonselective NSAIDs can be as high as three out of every 100 people. The risk is probably lower with nonacetylated salicylates such as salsalate. Salicylates in doses that are too high for you can make your ears ring and affect your hearing.

Rare: Bleeding from an ulcer, perforation of the bowel, liver problems, and kidney problems can occur. People who are allergic to aspirin and who have wheezing, a lumpy and itchy rash, and swelling of the tongue or face when they take aspirin are often allergic to other NSAIDs. Reye's syndrome is a very rare problem that caused liver failure and coma in children treated with aspirin for a viral illness. It virtually disappeared after the recommendation that aspirin should not be used in children, so other salicylates are also generally avoided in children.

Interactions with Other Drugs

Antacids: Antacids can decrease the effect of salicylates by increasing their excretion in the urine.

Warfarin *(Coumadin):* Salicylates can increase the anti-coagulant (anti–blood clotting) effect of warfarin in some people. If you are taking warfarin to prevent blood clots and you start taking a salicylate, you may need to have your blood monitored more frequently than usual, and your dose of warfarin may need to be changed. Nonacetylated salicylates do not affect platelet stickiness.

NSAIDs: A combination of two NSAIDs is avoided because it does not improve the control of inflammation but does increase the risk of side effects. But if someone on an NSAID needs aspirin to prevent a heart attack or stroke, then a low dose of aspirin is often prescribed with the other NSAID.

Methotrexate: Aspirin, other salicylates, and other NSAIDs can increase the concentrations of methotrexate, usually by a small amount. In rheumatology practice, with the low doses of methotrexate used, this interaction is seldom important and methotrexate is often prescribed with an NSAID for RA.

Lithium: Many NSAIDs can increase lithium levels. Lithium levels are usually monitored and the dose of lithium can be decreased if needed.

Diuretics ("water pills") or ACE (angiotensin converting enzyme) inhibitors—a family of drugs that lowers blood pressure: Many NSAIDs blunt the ability of these drugs to lower blood pressure.

Important Information

- Taking NSAIDs with food is a good idea and may protect you from indigestion, but it does not prevent peptic ulcers.
- Nonacetylated salicylates have little effect on platelet stickiness.
- One of the signs that you may be bleeding from the stomach is if you have pitch-black bowel movements. Bowel movements with altered blood, in addition to being black, are also often runny and very smelly. If this happens, contact your doctor immediately.

Common Dose Sizes

Capsule: 500 mg.
Tablet: 500 mg, 750 mg.

Usual Adult Doses

The usual adult dose of salsalate is 3 g a day split into two or three doses.

Comments

Nonacetylated salicylates are salicylates like aspirin, but their different chemical structure makes them behave more like COX-2 selective NSAIDs so that they have little effect on platelet stickiness and are kinder on the stomach. Some patients find that they are not as effective as other NSAIDs for controlling arthritis symptoms. Nonacetylated salicylates are a useful option for people who have stomach problems with NSAIDs or who are at high risk for NSAIDs causing stomach ulcers.

SANDIMMUNE (SEE CYCLOSPORINE)

SERTRALINE (*ZOLOFT;* SEE ***PROFILES OF COMMON ANTIDEPRESSANT DRUGS*** UNDER AMITRIPTYLINE)

SOLGANAL (SEE GOLD INJECTIONS)

SOMA (SEE CARISOPRODOL)

SUCRALFATE

Brand Name

Carafate.

Drug Family

Sucralfate belongs to the family of drugs used to treat peptic ulcers.

Families of Arthritis Problems Prescribed For

Sucralfate is used to treat peptic ulcers and to prevent damage to the stomach caused by NSAIDs.

How It Works

Sucralfate binds to damaged areas of the stomach, coats these areas, and protects them from stomach acid.

Avoid

Do not take sucralfate if you are allergic to it.

Take Precautions

• Sucralfate contains aluminum, which can accumulate in people with poor kidney function.

Side Effects

Sucralfate has very few side effects and is well tolerated.

Common: Constipation can be a problem in some people.

Interactions with Other Drugs

Many drugs: Sucralfate can bind to many drugs in the stomach so that they are not absorbed into your body. Delay taking your other medicines for two hours after you have taken sucralfate.

H_2-receptor antagonists (see CIMETIDINE) and proton pump inhibitors (see OMEPRAZOLE): Sucralfate needs acid in the stomach to be able to coat the damaged areas. These drugs stop the stomach from making acid and so block the effects of sucralfate.

Important Information

- Delay taking your other medicines for two hours after you have taken sucralfate.

Common Dose Sizes

Tablet: 1g.

Usual Adult Doses

The usual adult dose of sucralfate is 1 g four times a day to heal an ulcer and 1 g twice a day to protect the stomach.

Comments

There is more evidence showing that H_2-receptor antagonists (see CIMETIDINE) and proton pump inhibitors (see OMEPRAZOLE) heal peptic ulcers, so I prefer to use them. Some people find that sucralfate—one tablet dissolved in half a glass of water—used to "swish and spit" helps the pain caused by mouth ulcers.

SULFASALAZINE

Brand Names

Azulfidine, Azulfidine EN-tabs.

Sometimes Called

Salazopyrin, 5-aminosalicylic acid (5 ASA) + sulfapyridine.

Drug Family

Sulfasalazine is a disease-modifying antirheumatic drug (DMARD). It is a combination of a sulfonamide antibiotic and a salicylate that is not absorbed very well.

Families of Arthritis Problems Prescribed For

Sulfasalazine is used as a DMARD to treat RA. It is also used for other types of inflammatory arthritis such as juvenile rheumatoid arthritis, Reiter's syndrome, ankylosing spondylitis, and psoriatic arthritis. Sulfasalazine is often used to treat people with inflammatory bowel disease, whether they have arthritis with it or not.

How It Works

We are not sure exactly how sulfasalazine works. The antibiotic component is important, and it may be working by decreasing the bacteria that get into your bloodstream from the bowel.

Avoid

Do not take sulfasalazine if you are allergic to sulfonamides ("sulfa drugs") or if you are allergic to aspirin or other salicylates.

Take Precautions

• People who have inherited low levels of an enzyme called glucose-6 phosphate dehydrogenase (G-6PD) can break down their red blood cells when they take sulfasalazine. G-6PD deficiency is more common in certain ethnic groups (African, Mediterranean, East Asian). In people belonging to these ethnic groups, a blood test to check for G-6PD deficiency is sometimes done before sulfasalazine treatment is started.

• Your blood count will be monitored frequently, particularly when you begin treatment. Liver tests are usually checked from time to time.

Side Effects

Common: A rash and gastrointestinal symptoms are fairly common. Sulfasalazine can cause nausea, vomiting, diarrhea, and cramps but does not cause peptic ulcers, so people who cannot take aspirin or NSAIDs because of GI ulcers are okay with sulfasalazine. The GI side effects of sulfasalazine are not serious, but some people cannot take it because they find these side effects too bothersome.

Rare: A very low white blood cell count, a serious peeling skin rash, serious liver problems, drug-induced lupus, and skin sensitivity to sunlight are rare. Sulfasalazine can cause breakdown of red blood cells, called hemolysis, and anemia in people who are G-6PD deficient. This side effect is uncommon. In men, sulfasalazine can decrease the sperm count.

Interactions with Other Drugs

Warfarin *(Coumadin):* Sulfasalazine can increase the anticoagulant (anti–blood clotting) effect of warfarin in some people. If you are taking warfarin to prevent blood clots and you start taking sulfasalazine, you may need to have your blood monitored more frequently than usual, and your dose of warfarin may need to be changed.

Methotrexate: Sulfasalazine may increase the side effects of methotrexate. This does not seem to be a problem in practice, and the combination of these two DMARDs is often used (see Comments).

Important Information

- Make sure that you have the recommended blood tests done.
- If you develop a rash, stop taking the drug and contact your physician.
- Do not take more than the prescribed dose of sulfasalazine. Sulfasalazine needs to be taken regularly for it to work. Sulfasalazine does not control acute pain; it works as a DMARD by switching the inflammation off. There is no point in taking extra doses of sulfasalazine when you are hurting—in fact, it may be dangerous.
- Sulfasalazine can occasionally cause skin, urine, and contact lenses to have an orange-yellow color.
- Like most DMARDs, sulfasalazine works slowly, and it may be several weeks or even a couple of months before you see an improvement.

Common Dose Sizes

Tablets: 500 mg.
Tablet, enteric-coated: 500 mg.

Usual Adult Doses

The usual adult dose of sulfasalazine for arthritis-related problems is 2 or 3 g a day divided up into two or three doses.

I usually start with a low dose, such as 500 mg once or twice a day, and increase it if there are no side effects. The usual stable dose of sulfasalazine for most people is 2 g a day. Most physicians prescribe the enteric-coated preparation of sulfasalazine because it may cause fewer GI side effects.

Comments

The GI side effects of sulfasalazine are often worse soon after someone starts treatment. These seem to be less bothersome if you start with a low dose and work up. In RA sulfasalazine is an effective DMARD, and in some studies it is as good as methotrexate. Sulfasalazine is the most popular DMARD for RA in Europe. Sulfasalazine may have more nuisance side effects than methotrexate, but it has some advantages over methotrexate because it does not suppress the immune system, it does not cause methotrexate lung, and it does not cause liver scarring. Some rheumatologists think that methotrexate is more effective and, on average, better tolerated than sulfasalazine. Sulfasalazine is a useful alternative to methotrexate. More recently, combination treatment with methotrexate, sulfasalazine, and hydroxychloroquine was found to be helpful for some people whose RA was not controlled with a single DMARD.

In problems such as ankylosing spondylitis, sulfasalazine is more effective for treating swelling and inflammation of peripheral joints such as knees or wrists than it is for treating spine or back problems.

SULFINPYRAZONE

Brand Name

Anturane.

Drug Family

Sulfinpyrazone belongs to the family of drugs that lowers the uric acid level in your body.

Families of Arthritis Problems Prescribed For

Sulfinpyrazone is used to decrease the uric acid level in your body, and by doing this it prevents attacks of gout.

How It Works

Sulfinpyrazone is called a uricosuric drug because it gets rid of uric acid from your body by increasing the uric acid concentration in your urine.

Avoid

Do not take sulfinpyrazone if you are allergic to it or have poor kidney function. Sulfinpyrazone is avoided in people who have active peptic ulcers or who have had serious bone marrow problems.

Take Precautions

- A blood test is usually taken from time to time to check your uric acid level. The drop in the uric acid level after treatment can be a useful guide to how effective the treatment is.

Side Effects

Common: Gastrointestinal symptoms such as nausea and cramps are common; vomiting is less common.

Rare: A rash, itching, an allergic reaction, bringing on an attack of gout, bone marrow problems, liver problems, and kidney problems are rare.

Interactions with Other Drugs

Aspirin and other salicylates: Salicylates like aspirin can block the way sulfinpyrazone gets rid of uric acid in your urine.

Warfarin *(Coumadin):* Sulfinpyrazone can increase the anticoagulant (anti–blood clotting) effect of warfarin in some people. If you are taking warfarin to prevent blood clots and start taking sulfinpyrazone, you may need to have your blood monitored more frequently than usual, and your dose of warfarin may need to be changed.

Theophylline (*Theo-Dur* and many others): Sulfinpyrazone can decrease the blood levels of theophylline.

Verapamil *(Calan, Isoptin):* Sulfinpyrazone can decrease the blood levels of verapamil.

Important Information

- Sulfinpyrazone is taken regularly to prevent gout. Your risk for getting gout does not usually go away. To keep attacks of gout away, sulfinpyrazone often needs to be taken for many years, or indefinitely. Sulfinpyrazone may not completely prevent attacks of acute gout. If you have an attack of gout while you are taking sulfinpyrazone, remember that sulfinpyrazone has no effect on the pain and swelling of the acute attack. A common mistake people make is to take their sulfinpyrazone only when they get an attack of gout.
- Drink plenty of fluids. Sulfinpyrazone increases the uric acid concentrations in your urine, so keeping your urine dilute will decrease your risk of getting uric acid kidney stones.

Common Dose Sizes

Tablet: 100 mg.
Capsule: 200 mg.

Usual Adult Doses

The usual adult dose of sulfinpyrazone is 100 mg or 200 mg twice a day, up to a maximum of 800 mg a day.

SULINDAC

Brand Name

Clinoril.

Drug Family

Sulindac belongs to the nonsteroidal anti-inflammatory drug (NSAID) family. There are two big groups of NSAIDs, divided by whether they inhibit both cyclo-oxygenase (COX) enzymes, COX-1 and COX-2, or are more selective for COX-2. Sulindac inhibits both COX-1 and COX-2.

Families of Arthritis Problems Prescribed For

NSAIDs are used to treat all kinds of pain and inflammation, whether they affect the joints or not. NSAIDs are used to treat many kinds of arthritis problems, such as RA, osteoarthritis, and bursitis. NSAIDs decrease pain and inflammation, but they do not change the progression of arthritis.

How It Works

Most NSAIDs inhibit the enzymes COX-1 and COX-2. Inhibiting these cyclo-oxygenase enzymes decreases the formation of chemicals called prostaglandins. Decreasing the prostaglandins made by COX-2 is anti-inflammatory, which is usually why we use NSAIDs. NSAIDs that inhibit COX-1 make platelets in your blood less sticky. COX-1 also protects the stomach from ulcers, so blocking COX-1 may be why most NSAIDs increase the risk of peptic ulcers.

Avoid

Do not take sulindac if you are allergic to it. People who have had a serious allergic reaction (swelling of the face and tongue, and wheezing) to one NSAID can have the same reaction to others. People with asthma or nasal polyps are more likely to be allergic to NSAIDs. NSAIDs are avoided if someone has an active peptic ulcer or is pregnant.

Take Precautions

- NSAIDs can cause fluid retention and can worsen heart failure and high blood pressure.
- Some people are at higher risk for peptic ulcers caused by NSAIDs. Risk factors are being older than 65 years, having had a previous peptic ulcer, having had a previous bleeding ulcer, and taking a corticosteroid. In people who have a higher risk for peptic ulcers caused by NSAIDs, most rheumatologists would avoid NSAIDs, if possible. If this is not possible, then prescribing misoprostol (see MISOPROSTOL—*Cytotec*) or a proton pump inhibitor (see OMEPRAZOLE—*Prilosec*) to protect against peptic ulcers caused by NSAIDs is an option. Another option is to use a COX-2 selective NSAID such as ROFECOXIB *(Vioxx)* or CELECOXIB *(Celebrex)*. None of these choices is foolproof, and peptic ulcers can still develop.
- NSAIDs have to be used carefully in people who have asthma or liver or kidney problems.
- If you are taking NSAIDs regularly, blood tests will be done from time to time to check your blood count (in case you are losing blood slowly from an ulcer that you may not know about), your creatinine (for kidney function), and liver enzymes. People taking diuretics ("water pills") or ACE (angiotensin converting enzyme) inhibitors—a family of drugs that lowers blood pressure—and people with diabetes, heart failure, or existing kidney problems are more likely to have kidney problems caused by NSAIDs. These people may need more frequent blood tests to check their kidney function.

Side Effects

See NSAIDs.

Interactions with Other Drugs

See NSAIDs.

Important Information

- Taking NSAIDs with food is a good idea and may protect you from indigestion, but it does not prevent peptic ulcers.
- To minimize your gastrointestinal risks, use the lowest effective dose of an NSAID.
- One of the signs that you may be bleeding from the stomach is if you have pitch-black bowel movements. Bowel movements with altered blood, in addition to being black, are also often runny and very smelly. If this happens, contact your doctor immediately.

Common Dose Sizes

Tablet: 150 mg, 200 mg.

Usual Adult Doses

The usual adult dose of sulindac is 150 mg or 200 mg twice a day.

Comments

See NSAIDs.

Sulindac may be slightly safer than other NSAIDs in people with kidney problems, but this is controversial.

SYNVISC (HYLAN GF 20) (SEE HYALURONAN INJECTIONS)

TACROLIMUS

Brand Name

Prograf.

Sometimes Called

FK506.

Drug Family

Tacrolimus is an antirejection drug that is used to prevent rejection after someone has had an organ transplant. It is very similar to cyclosporine in how it works and its side effects.

Families of Arthritis Problems Prescribed For

Tacrolimus is not approved by the FDA for the treatment of any rheumatic problem. It is being tested as a disease-modifying antirheumatic drug (DMARD) for RA, but the studies have not been completed.

Comments

Tacrolimus is not yet used to treat rheumatic problems, but it is a drug that you may hear or read about. In the next few years we will know if tacrolimus offers advantages over cyclosporine for treating some arthritis problems. Tacrolimus works in a way very similar to the way cyclosporine does, has very similar side effects, and also interacts with the same drugs that cyclosporine does (see CYCLOSPORINE).

TEARS, ARTIFICIAL (SEE ARTIFICIAL TEARS)

TETRACYCLINES (SEE MINOCYCLINE)

THALIDOMIDE

Brand Name

Thalomid.

Drug Family

Thalidomide is a sleeping tablet that was taken off the market in 1961, when it was realized that it caused birth defects. Thalidomide also alters the immune response.

Families of Arthritis Problems Prescribed For

Recently thalidomide has been tested (under strict controls) for problems such as mouth ulcers in people with HIV, mouth and genital ulcers in people with Behçet's disease (an uncommon problem that can cause mouth and genital ulcers and eye and joint problems), and skin problems in lupus that have not responded to other treatments.

How It Works

It is not clear how thalidomide changes the immune response, but it decreases formation of tumor necrosis factor (TNF) and also decreases the formation of new blood vessels (angiogenesis).

Avoid

Do not take thalidomide if you are pregnant, wish to become pregnant, or plan to make someone else pregnant. Do not take thalidomide unless you are prepared to use two reliable methods of birth control. Do not take thalidomide if you are allergic to it.

Take Precautions

• Thalidomide will be prescribed only as an "investigational drug" with very strict controls. You will be given written information about thalidomide and may be asked to watch a video about it. You will sign an informed consent document stating that you understand the risks of treatment, and you will have to provide information to a national registry that is tracking the side effects of thalidomide.

• Never take anyone else's thalidomide.

• Never share your thalidomide with anyone else.

• Your physicians will make absolutely sure that you are not pregnant before you start thalidomide.

• If you can bear children, you must make absolutely sure that you do not become pregnant while you are taking thalidomide by using two reliable birth-control methods for four weeks before, during, and continuing for at least four weeks after you have finished treatment with thalidomide. The effects of birth-control pills can be reduced by many other medicines such as antibiotics and antiseizure medicines. If you are taking medicines that reduce the effects of birth-control pills, you may have to use two other methods of birth control or avoid sex.

• Men taking thalidomide, even if they have had a vasectomy, must use latex condoms because some thalidomide may be in semen.

• Your blood count will be checked from time to time to make sure that thalidomide is not decreasing your white blood cell count.

Side Effects

Common: Thalidomide causes serious birth defects. Nerve damage, which can be painful, severe, and permanent, can occur. Other side effects are sleepiness, constipation, a rash, headaches, and fluid retention (edema). You can feel dizzy if you get up suddenly after you have been sitting or lying down.

Less common: Thalidomide can cause a drop in your white cell count.

Interactions with Other Drugs

There is very little information about drug combinations that include thalidomide.

Alcohol and other sedatives: These increase the sedative effects of thalidomide.

Important Information

- Your doctor will monitor you regularly for nerve damage. But if you notice numbness, "pins and needles," tingling, or burning of your hands or feet, these may be signs of nerve damage and you should tell your doctor.
- If you miss your menstrual period while you are taking thalidomide, contact your doctor immediately.
- Thalidomide can cause drowsiness and affect your concentration during driving and performing other tasks.
- Keep thalidomide away from children.

Common Dose Sizes

Capsule: 50 mg.

Usual Adult Doses

The usual adult dose of thalidomide is 50 to 300 mg a day. Higher doses cause more side effects.

Comments

The problem with using thalidomide for arthritis-related problems is that even if it works, it only suppresses the problem temporarily, and the problem comes back when thalidomide is stopped. Thalidomide is not a good drug to use for a long time because of the risk of permanent nerve damage, and for many people the potential risks outweigh the benefits. New drugs similar to thalidomide are being developed that do not cause nerve damage or birth defects.

TOLECTIN (SEE TOLMETIN)

TOLMETIN

Brand Name

Tolectin.

Drug Family

Tolmetin belongs to the nonsteroidal anti-inflammatory drug (NSAID) family. There are two big groups of NSAIDs, divided by whether they inhibit both cyclo-oxygenase (COX) enzymes, COX-1 and COX-2, or are more selective for COX-2. Tolmetin inhibits both COX-1 and COX-2.

Families of Arthritis Problems Prescribed For

NSAIDs are used to treat all kinds of pain and inflammation, whether they affect the joints or not. NSAIDs are used to treat many kinds of arthritis problems, such as RA, osteoarthritis, and bursitis. NSAIDs decrease pain and inflammation, but they do not change the progression of arthritis.

How It Works

Most NSAIDs inhibit the enzymes COX-1 and COX-2. Inhibiting these cyclo-oxygenase enzymes decreases the formation of chemicals called prostaglandins. Decreasing the prostaglandins made by COX-2 is anti-inflammatory, which is usually why we use NSAIDs. NSAIDs that inhibit COX-1 make platelets in your blood less sticky. COX-1 also protects the stomach from ulcers, so blocking COX-1 may be why the most NSAIDs increase the risk of peptic ulcers.

Avoid

Do not take tolmetin if you are allergic to it. People who have had a serious allergic reaction (swelling of the face and tongue, and wheezing) to one NSAID can have the same reaction with others. People with asthma or nasal polyps are more likely to be allergic to NSAIDs. NSAIDs are avoided if someone has an active peptic ulcer or is pregnant.

Take Precautions

- NSAIDs can cause fluid retention and can worsen heart failure and high blood pressure.
- Some people are at higher risk for peptic ulcers caused by NSAIDs. Risk factors are being older than 65 years, having had a previous peptic ulcer, having had a previous bleeding ulcer, and taking a corticosteroid. In people who have a higher risk for peptic ulcers caused by NSAIDs, most rheumatologists would avoid NSAIDs, if possible. If this is not possible, then prescribing misoprostol (see MISOPROSTOL—*Cytotec*) or a proton pump inhibitor (see OMEPRAZOLE—*Prilosec*) to protect against peptic ulcers caused by NSAIDs is an option. Another option is to use a COX-2 selective NSAID such as ROFECOXIB *(Vioxx)* or CELECOXIB *(Celebrex)*. None of these choices is foolproof, and peptic ulcers can still develop.
- NSAIDs have to be used carefully in people who have asthma or liver or kidney problems.
- If you are taking NSAIDs regularly, blood tests will be done from time to time to check your blood count (in case you are losing blood slowly from an ulcer that you may not know about), your creatinine (for kidney function), and liver

enzymes. People taking diuretics ("water pills") or ACE (angiotensin converting enzyme) inhibitors—a family of drugs that lowers blood pressure—and people with diabetes, heart failure, or existing kidney problems are more likely to have kidney problems caused by NSAIDs. These people may need more frequent blood tests to check their kidney function.

Side Effects.

See NSAIDs.

Interactions with Other Drugs

See NSAIDs.

Important Information

- Taking NSAIDs with food is a good idea and may protect you from indigestion, but it does not prevent peptic ulcers.
- To minimize your gastrointestinal risks, use the lowest effective dose of an NSAID.
- One of the signs that you may be bleeding from the stomach is if you have pitch-black bowel movements. Bowel movements with altered blood, in addition to being black, are also often runny and very smelly. If this happens, contact your doctor immediately.

Common Dose Sizes

Tablet: 200 mg, 400 mg, 600 mg.

Usual Adult Doses

The usual adult dose of tolmetin is 600 mg to 1,800 mg a day split into three or four doses.

Comments

See NSAIDs.

TORADOL (SEE KETOROLAC)

TRAMADOL

Brand Name
Ultram.

Drug Family
Tramadol is a narcotic analgesic (painkiller).

Families of Arthritis Problems Prescribed For
Tramadol is used for moderate to severe pain, whatever the cause. Narcotic analgesics are usually only prescribed for pain that is not controlled by acetaminophen alone or an NSAID alone. Narcotics do not affect inflammation.

How It Works
Narcotics decrease pain by acting through specific receptors in the brain. Tramadol may have some painkilling effects that are not due to its narcotic actions.

Avoid
Do not take tramadol if you are allergic to it. Real allergic reactions are rare, but a lot of people get side effects such as nausea or feeling "spacy" from tramadol. Avoid tramadol if you have had an addiction problem.

Take Precautions

- Do not drink alcohol while you are taking narcotics.
- There is a risk of becoming addicted to narcotics. Tramadol is less likely to cause addiction than some stronger narcotics. Take the tablets only for pain. If possible, limit the

dose and how long you take them. One physician should be responsible for all your narcotic prescriptions.

• Caution is needed in people who have poor liver or kidney function or seizures.

Side Effects

Side effects are common with tramadol, but they are usually mild. People vary in their sensitivity to different narcotics. People who cannot take preparations that contain tramadol, for example, may be able to tolerate another preparation containing codeine, and vice versa.

Common: Nausea, headache, itching, vomiting, constipation, poor appetite, dizziness, lightheadedness or feeling "spacy," and sleepiness are common but not serious.

Less common: An allergic reaction with a rash, hives, or asthma is rare. Confusion, seizures, feeling nervous or agitated, sleeping badly, feeling "high," addictive behavior to try and get higher doses of narcotic to feel good rather than to control pain are uncommon but do occur.

Interactions with Other Drugs

Any other sedative drug: Narcotics make people sleepy, and an overdose can make people unconscious and stop their breathing. Combining a narcotic with another sedative drug, such as alcohol, is dangerous.

Antidepressants: The risk of seizures is increased if tramadol is combined with antidepressants (see AMITRIPTYLINE).

Quinidine (*Quinaglute* and many others): The blood levels of tramadol are increased by quinidine, and you may need smaller doses.

Cimetidine *(Tagamet):* The blood levels of tramadol are increased by cimetidine, and you may need smaller doses.

Important Information

- Don't take more than the prescribed dose.
- Don't drink alcohol while you are taking narcotic painkillers.
- Narcotics can cause drowsiness and affect your concentration when driving and performing other tasks.
- Tramadol is a narcotic and can be addictive (see Comments).
- Narcotics are dangerous in overdose. Keep them away from children.

Common Dose Sizes

Tablet: 50 mg.

Usual Adult Doses

The usual adult dose of tramadol is 50 mg to 100 mg every four to six hours, if needed, to control pain, up to a maximum of 400 mg a day.

Comments

There is some controversy about how narcotic analgesics should be used to control chronic "benign" pain, meaning chronic pain not caused by cancer. This is particularly true of the strong narcotics, such as morphine, but to a lesser extent is also true for weaker narcotics such as codeine, hydrocodone, and tramadol. Some physicians think that the risk of addiction and abuse is high and limit narcotic prescriptions to short periods, such as a few days, in all patients. Others are less rigid and believe that these analgesics can make life bearable for some people with chronic arthritis pain that cannot be controlled by other strategies. For example, I find them helpful to control pain at night in some people with severe osteoarthritis pain who cannot take NSAIDs because of their side effects. Most rheumatologists do not prescribe narcotics for fibromyalgia because they are not particularly helpful, and they can worsen the sleep disturbance.

Addiction to tramadol is rarely a problem if it is used to control pain. A clue to addictive behavior is if you are trying to get bigger doses of the drug and are not using the bigger doses to control pain. The risk of addiction is higher in people who themselves, or whose family members, have had an addiction problem (alcohol or drugs). I have a few rules for my patients about narcotic prescriptions.

1. Use the tablets only for pain, not to feel good.
2. If you don't have pain, don't take them.
3. Get all your narcotic prescriptions from one doctor and from one pharmacy.
4. Escalating the dose can be an early sign of a problem.
5. Never sell, swap, or hoard tablets.
6. If you are in the position of wanting to fool doctors or do illegal things such as forging signatures to get narcotic prescriptions, things are way out of control and you need to speak with your physician about getting help.

Tramadol is sometimes promoted as a non-narcotic analgesic, but it is a narcotic. The risk of addiction may be smaller than with other narcotics, but it should still be treated with respect. The potential to cause seizures with antidepressants limits its use. On average, tramadol is no better than other weaker narcotic analgesics such as codeine. People vary a lot, and some people find that tramadol suits them better than codeine or other weaker narcotic analgesics.

TRAZODONE (*DESYREL;* SEE ***PROFILES OF COMMON ANTIDEPRESSANT DRUGS*** UNDER AMITRIPTYLINE)

TRICYCLIC ANTIDEPRESSANTS (SEE AMITRIPTYLINE)

TRILISATE (SEE CHOLINE MAGNESIUM SALICYLATE)

TUMS (SEE CALCIUM)

TYLENOL (SEE ACETAMINOPHEN)

TYLENOL #3 (SEE ACETAMINOPHEN + NARCOTICS)

TYLOX (SEE ACETAMINOPHEN + NARCOTICS)

ULTRAM (SEE TRAMADOL)

VENLAFAXINE (*EFFEXOR*) (SEE ***PROFILES OF COMMON ANTIDEPRESSANT DRUGS*** UNDER AMITRIPTYLINE)

VICODIN (SEE ACETAMINOPHEN + NARCOTICS)

VIOXX (SEE ROFECOXIB)

VOLTAREN (SEE DICLOFENAC)

ZANTAC (RANITIDINE; SEE *PROFILES OF COMMON* H_2*-RECEPTOR ANTAGONIST DRUGS* UNDER CIMETIDINE)

ZOLPIDEM

Brand Name
Ambien.

Drug Family
Zolpidem is a sleeping pill. It has no effect on arthritis.

Families of Arthritis Problems Prescribed For
Zolpidem is used to improve sleep, sometimes in people with fibromyalgia.

How It Works
Zolpidem binds to the same receptors in the brain that drugs such as diazepam *(Valium)* and other benzodiazepines bind to, and it causes sleepiness.

Avoid
Do not take zolpidem if you are allergic to it.

Take Precautions
- Zolpidem may cause you to be sleepy and may affect your ability to drive or to operate machinery.

Side Effects
Common: Sleepiness is common, and sometimes people still feel "hung-over" the next day. Zolpidem can cause headache.

Less common: Most people get sleepy when they take zolpidem, but some people find the opposite—that it stimulates them and keeps them awake. Dizziness, an allergic reaction, confusion, and forgetfulness can occur.

Interactions with Other Drugs

Alcohol and other sedatives: These increase the sedative effects of zolpidem.

Important Information

- Avoid alcohol and antidepressants while you are taking zolpidem.

Common Dose Sizes

Tablets: 5 mg, 10 mg.

Usual Adult Doses

The dose of zolpidem is 10 mg before bedtime. In older people 5 mg is used.

Comments

As is true for most sleeping pills, it is best not to use zolpidem regularly, every night, for long periods. One of the advantages of zolpidem over the benzodiazepine family of drugs is that it is not addictive.

ZORPRIN (SEE ASPIRIN)

ZOSTRIX (SEE CAPSAICIN)

ZYLOPRIM (SEE ALLOPURINOL)

GLOSSARY OF FREQUENTLY USED ABBREVIATIONS AND ACRONYMS

DEXA—dual energy X-ray absorptiometry
DMARD—disease-modifying antirheumatic drug
GI—gastrointestinal
IV—intravenous
JRA—juvenile rheumatoid arthritis
NSAID—nonsteroidal anti-inflammatory drug
OA—osteoarthritis
RA—rheumatoid arthritis
SERMs—selective estrogen receptor modulators
SLE—systemic lupus erythematosus

INDEX

NOTE: **Bold** page numbers refer to primary discussion of the drug. Names in parentheses following drug names are brand names.

ABOUT THE AUTHOR

Dr. Michael Stein is both a practicing rheumatologist and a clinical pharmacologist. This background provides him with practical experience in treating many hundreds of patients with arthritis, and also special expertise in evaluating the drugs that are used to treat arthritis. Dr. Stein graduated from the University of Cape Town, South Africa, in 1978, did his internship in New Zealand, and then worked for many years in Zimbabwe, sometimes as the only rheumatologist in that country. He came to the United States in 1990. He has published more than ninety scientific papers, book chapters, and editorials in the medical literature and is a recognized authority in the area of drug therapy for rheumatic diseases.

Dr. Stein is currently an Associate Professor of Medicine at a large academic medical center where he treats patients with rheumatic problems, teaches, and conducts research.